AF734779

Understanding the institutional dynamics of South Africa's response to the HIV/Aids pandemic

Ann Strode

Kitty Barrett Grant

Institute for Democracy in South Africa (Idasa)
Cnr Prinsloo & Visagie Streets
PO Box 56950
Arcadia 0007
Pretoria, RSA
E-mail: Kondwani@idasa.org.za or Mary@idasa.org.za
Tel: 27-12-3920500• Fax: 27-12-3202414/5

ISBN 1-919-798-66-8

Cover design: Magenta Media
Text design/DTP: Page Arts cc
Content edit: Mary Caesar & Kondwani Chirambo
Copy edit: Laurie Rose-Innes and Moira Levy

This publication has been produced with the assistance of the Ford Foundation. Its contents are the sole responsibility of Idasa and in no way reflect the views of the Ford Foundation.

Idasa is an independent public interest organisation committed to promoting a sustainable democracy in South Africa and elsewhere by building democratic institutions, educating citizens and advocating social justice. The evolution of Idasa's mission and its programmes tells the story of the transition to democracy in South Africa, and the challenges of democratisation that continue to confront us. Its work in democracy, governance and HIV/Aids covers Southern Africa and Africa in general.

Understanding the institutional dynamics of South Africa's response to the HIV/Aids pandemic

Ann Strode
Kitty Barrett Grant

2004

About the authors

Ann Elaine Strode, LLM, LLB and BA in religious studies and political science, University of Natal, is a senior lecturer at the School of Law, University of KwaZulu-Natal, Pietermaritzburg. She jointly co-ordinated the Department of Health's HIV/Aids Law and Human Rights Programme within the National HIV/Aids and STD Directorate with Ms Barrett Grant. Prior to this, she was the regional director for Lawyers for Human Rights, and has been a member of the University of KwaZulu-Natal's HIV/Aids vaccine and ethics research group. She has consulted extensively for international and donor agencies in various capacities. Ann was the principal researcher on the Idasa-GAP Sanac study.

Kitty Barrett Grant, BA (Wits) LLB (Unisa), is an admitted attorney with extensive experience in the field of HIV/Aids law and human rights. Between 1997 and 2000 she and Ms Strode jointly co-ordinated the Department of Health's Law and Human Rights Programme for the National HIV/Aids and STD Directorate. At present, she consults to a wide range of organisations, including the government, NGOs and international agencies, on areas of the law relating to HIV and Aids, with a particular focus on the development of HIV/Aids workplace policies. Kitty was the assistant researcher on the Idasa-GAP Sanac study.

The Governance and Aids Programme (GAP) staff

Kondwani Chirambo	*Programme Manager*
Vasanthie Naicker	*Programme Administrator*
Mary Caesar	*Research Facilitator*
Diana Naburi-Koikai	*Research Facilitator*
Marietjie Myburg	*Regional Media Co-ordinator*
Shaila Gupta	*Researcher*
Beate Jaschik	*Intern*

Table of Contents

List of tables

Acronyms

ANC	African National Congress
ARVs	Anti-retrovirals
ATIC	Aids Training and Information Centre
CCM	Country co-ordinating mechanism, a term used by the GFATM to describe the body that co-ordinates the programmes that have received funding within a state
DoH	Department of Health
ECI (KZN)	Enhancing Care Initiative (KwaZulu-Natal)
GFATM	Global Fund for Aids, Tuberculosis and Malaria
IDC	Inter-departmental Committee on HIV/Aids
IMC	Inter-ministerial Committee
MEC	Members of the Executive Council (i.e. Provincial Cabinet Ministers)
MinMec	Meeting of MECs
Nacosa	National Aids Co-ordinating Committee of South Africa
Napwa	National Association of People Living with HIV and Aids
Nepad	New Partnership for Africa's Development
NGO	Non-governmental organisation
PAC	Provincial Aids Council
PLWA	Person(s) living with HIV or Aids
SADC	Southern African Development Community
Sanac	South African National Aids Council
TAC	Treatment Action Campaign
UAC	Uganda Aids Commission

Acknowledgements

We acknowledge with thanks the continued support of the **Ford Foundation** to Idasa's Governance and Aids Programme (GAP), which has led to the materialisation of this report. The research report is part of a four-country study involving researchers in Namibia, Mozambique, South Africa and Zimbabwe. The study was made possible by the co-operation of stakeholders in government and civil society sectors who agreed to be interviewed on their perceptions, assessments and involvement in the institutional response to the Aids pandemic in South Africa. The study was conducted in the spirit of contributing to strengthening the partnerships between the state and non-state actors. It has to be emphasised that this is not an official evaluation of the South African National Aids Council (Sanac).

The project was co-ordinated by Mary Caesar, the research facilitator on GAP, who worked closely with the consultants in all four countries. These studies were initiated in mid-2003 as part of a broader scheme to understand more comprehensively the nature of the response and strategic partnerships constructed to deal with the Aids pandemic. Inevitably, the study looked at the weaknesses and strengths of Aids council structures and their place in the highly complex political environment that conditions the level of commitment and leadership.

The draft report of the South Africa study (along with the Mozambique and Zimbabwe reports) was shared with a wider group of stakeholders in South Africa drawn from the Department of Health, provincial government structures, the SADC Health Sector Co-ordinating Unit, the Joint United Nations Programme on HIV/Aids, the United Nations Development Programme, civil society, the private sector and aid agencies at a round-table meeting held in Pretoria on 27 November 2003.

Ultimately, the studies are designed to contribute to the exchange of best practices on the governance of HIV/Aids in the Southern African region and to strengthening multi-sectoral responses.

I wish to finally acknowledge the contribution of all of the staff of GAP, particularly Vasanthie Naicker, the programme administrator, who made the necessary logistical arrangements for the research teams to perform their work, and Diana Naburi-Koikai for the final touches to the document. If we have failed to acknowledge others whose valuable input we benefited from, we do sincerely apologise.

Kondwani Chirambo
Manager
Governance and AIDS Programme

1 Introduction

Kondwani Chirambo

Idasa's Governance and Aids Programme (GAP) seeks to create awareness around the potential impact of the HIV/Aids pandemic on governance processes in Africa. The programme recognises that Aids is a highly complex pandemic of crisis proportions that is impacting on institutions and participation of citizens in political and economic life, with serious implications for governance. It stresses the need for effective governance of the pandemic, based on strong relationships between the state, civil society and the private sector in mobilising resources and implementing programmes. In this regard, the programme aims to build consensus and reformulate the vision on how to deal with this disaster. GAP uses research outputs as an advocacy tool to influence policy and programmes through key stakeholders such as lawmakers, government representatives, Aids councils and civil society. This could contribute to the institutionalisation of holistic HIV/Aids strategies.

Defining governance

GAP subscribes to the definition of governance as: "a set of values, policies and institutions by which a society manages its economic, political and social processes at all levels through interaction among government, civil society and private sector".[1]

Values or principles

Although there may be no global harmony on what forms the core values of governance, there is general agreement that the manner in which the state, society and economy interact is vital for development. There is also increasing evidence of emerging consensus on certain core elements of governance that suggest a movement from state-focused definitions of the concept. For instance, Olowu and Sako (2002: 18,19) explain that in the perspective typified by development agencies such as the United Nations Development Programme (UNDP), "governance comprises the mechanisms, processes, and institutions through which citizens and groups articulate their interests, exercise their rights, meet their obligations and mediate their conflicts".[2]

The World Bank views governance "as the process and institutions by which authority in a country is exercised". The Bank conceives the process of governance to include how "governments are selected, held accountable, monitored and replaced".[3] Its working definition, designed perhaps to suit its regulation and evaluation of relations with member states, also speaks to the capacity of governments to manage resources and "respect of the institutions and rule of law that govern economic and social interaction". Still, the components of governance, as seen through the lens of the Bank, embrace the presence of a vibrant civil society, accountability, control of corruption (or transparency), political stability and the quality of regulatory frameworks.

Closer to home, the African Union's New Partnership for Africa's Development (Nepad) also subscribes to "global standards" of political governance and democracy. Its democracy and political governance initiative pledges to act in line with "the principles of democracy".[4] Nepad's founding vision statement cites transparency, accountability, integrity, respect for human rights and promotion of the rule of law as being cardinal to bolstering political and economic governance, leading to development and eradication of poverty.[5] In all of the current discourses on governance, emphasis is laid on the rule of law, participation, accountability and especially the promotion of human rights.

Therefore, although the principles or values of governance are not unanimously accepted worldwide, they do in fact seem to achieve the closest possible approximation of universality when a rights-based approach is adopted. At least 171 member states of the United Nations (UN) have reaffirmed their dedication to the Universal Declaration of Human Rights (UDHR). More than half of the UN members are state-parties to all six principal human rights treaties that emphasise citizen's rights and freedoms and by implication the state's responsibility to achieving them.[6] Put another way, states that have ratified the UDHR and instruments such as the International Covenant on Civil and Political Rights (ICCPR) in principle subscribe to the notion that the citizen is entitled to good governance as "a public good".[7]

This, among other things, means that it is the state's responsibility to create conditions that enable all its citizens – in particular the marginalised – to avoid consignment to premature mortality, starvation and undernourishment and that all people enjoy rights that serve as a medium for participation in the political process.[8] The conduct of public affairs should hence be seen to measure up to the values that best speak to a rights-compliant society.

Overall, the emergent common values of governance include *accountability of leadership*, *participation* and *representation*[9] of all sections of society in decision-making processes; *transparency*, so the affairs of state are conducted in an honest and forthright manner; *equality*, particularly *gender equality and equity*,[10] to ensure that prejudices are outlawed; and upholding *the rule of law* and respecting *human rights*. Other values are *responsiveness* and the *commitment of the leadership* to addressing political, economic and social needs as an obligation. Governance may hence be deemed "good" when it meets the aspirations of its citizens underpinned by the stipulated global values.

Viewing governance from this global human rights prism should assist Africa's Peer Review Mechanism (APRM) to be effective and internationally accepted;[11] it does certainly assist development agencies, non-governmental organisations and practitioners of all descriptions to develop indicators and thereby measure governance.[12]

Defining the values of governance on the basis of international human rights approaches is also extremely relevant to the management of the HIV/Aids pandemic, particularly as it relates to key issues such as stigma, discrimination[13] and access to treatment, care and support.

Broad domains of governance

The literature indicates that the concept and process of governance is all encapsulating and may be divided into four main domains:

- political governance;
- institutional governance;
- economic governance; and
- corporate and global governance.

Political governance

Political and institutional structures and processes constitute the nucleus of governance, indicating the prolific role of the political system and institutional setting in establishing the quality of governance. It is argued that the political and institutional environment shape and determine the extent of human rights – civil and political rights, economic and social rights – in their entirety.[14]

The core elements of political governance include:

- basic political rights (e.g. the right to belong to an association or political movement of one's choice);
- freedom of expression;
- competitive and free and fair elections;
- supremacy of the law;
- broad-based participation in local governance and community forums; and
- an independent judiciary.

A weakness in the political governance of a country could lead to disregard for pressing national concerns such as HIV/Aids in preference for greater investment in the military or presidential travel and privileges, for instance. Or it could lead to the failure of citizens infected and affected by HIV/Aids to access justice due to unresponsive judicial mechanisms. Worse still, poor political governance might compromise the ability of citizens to demonstrate against bad policy due to arbitrary statutory impositions. The absence of competition in the political system will by itself dilute the strength of the voices that demand action on matters of public interest.

Institutional governance

The institutional dimension refers to administrative structures and processes through which policy design, implementation, monitoring and evaluation are undertaken. These need to be all-inclusive rather than state-centred. In other words, there must be channels for wider consultation with civil society (such as through community forums). There must be channels of influence through which an independent public service could motivate the political leadership on the need for alternative policies.[15]

Economic governance

Economic governance refers to the processes of decision-making that directly or indirectly impact on the economic activities of a country and its relationship with other economies. This domain of governance includes the institutions that formulate, implement, monitor and evaluate development policies, and include government departments and the central bank. The World Bank, International Monetary Fund (IMF) and other creditor and donor agencies, and supranational formations, are all international players in the area of economic governance.[16] This aspect of governance testifies to the fact that most countries, particularly developing counties, are not entirely in control of their internal political and economic affairs. They must, for instance, adhere to templates for development prescribed by the IMF, the World Bank and other Western donors. It may be argued that this in itself might have an impact on what issues – including HIV/Aids – are prioritised in the national budget.

Among other things, economic governance is meant to:

- ensure that people have access to employment, education and health facilities (development experts would say that people should have their *choices expanded* and be able to enjoy *long healthy lives*);
- ensure wider participation of citizens in the development process (as economic growth does not automatically translate into benefits for all); and
- ensure that there is empowerment (or expand people's capabilities), equity (increasing opportunities that are not necessarily income-centric) and sustainability (meeting the needs of the present generation without jeopardising posterity – in short, the needs of a future generation should be reflected in existing policies).[17]

Corporate and global governance

Corporate governance is formed largely by the institutional and legal framework in which firms operate; this includes the arbitration mechanisms between boards of directors and trade unions. It does not ignore the bigger picture – the global environment conditioned by trans-national companies, which usually go unregulated by states due to the complex nature of the relationships.[18] The essence of corporate governance should be that organised business concerns work in concert with civil society and the state in moulding effective governance in society.

Because HIV/Aids is so complex as to threaten not only the productive members of society, but the capacity of the very institutions through which governance is to be achieved, it is imperative that a broad-based approach to the pandemic is adopted. Multi-sector, multi-level responses have been instituted in most countries in Africa but the internal dynamics of the institutional arrangements that have been set-up are often not sufficiently lubricated to meet the challenge of Aids and the related crises of poverty. Not only is political leadership required, a total mobilisation of cross-sectoral stakeholders is called for in the identification and prioritisation of key areas of intervention, and in the marshalling of resources and implementation of programmes. It is clear to us that the immensity of the problems of underdevelopment, exacerbated by the advent of Aids, require that the relationship between the state and non-state actors in leading development be strong and effective.

The greater involvement of non-state actors not only increases capacity, but potentially adds to efficiency in delivering services in all respects. It may be assumed hence that *good* governance in all domains would lead to economic progress and specifically to human development – poverty reduction, better education, employment opportunities and reasonably long healthy lives – with or without HIV/Aids.

2 Country profile

Geographic location

South Africa is the southernmost country in Africa. It is a member of the Southern African Development Community (SADC) and its neighbours are Botswana, Lesotho, Mozambique, Namibia, Swaziland and Zimbabwe.

Population

The 1996 census reported a population of 40 million people. Statistics South Africa reported in 2001 that the population had grown to 44 million people, of whom 23 million were women.

The population is made up of a number of different ethnic groups, with the Nguni people comprising two-thirds of the population. Other groups include the Sotho-Tswana people, the Tsonga, the Venda, Afrikaners, English, coloureds, and Indians.[19]

Political system

Since 1994 South Africa's new political order is enshrined in a constitutional democracy. The Constitution[20] is supreme, and the executive, legislature and judiciary must act in accordance with it. Fundamental human rights are protected within the Bill of Rights in the Constitution.

South Africa has a quasi-federal system, with legislative power shared between the National Assembly, National Council of Provinces and provincial legislatures.

HIV and Aids epidemics (and deaths)

In South Africa, as in most developing countries, the HIV and Aids epidemics have been well established for 20 years or more. Based on an antenatal survey completed in October 2000, 24.5 per cent of all pregnant women in South Africa are HIV positive; this enables us to project that 4.8 million South Africans are infected with HIV. Worryingly, nearly 20 per cent of all 15–49 year olds are infected.[21]

Table 1: HIV prevalence in South Africa

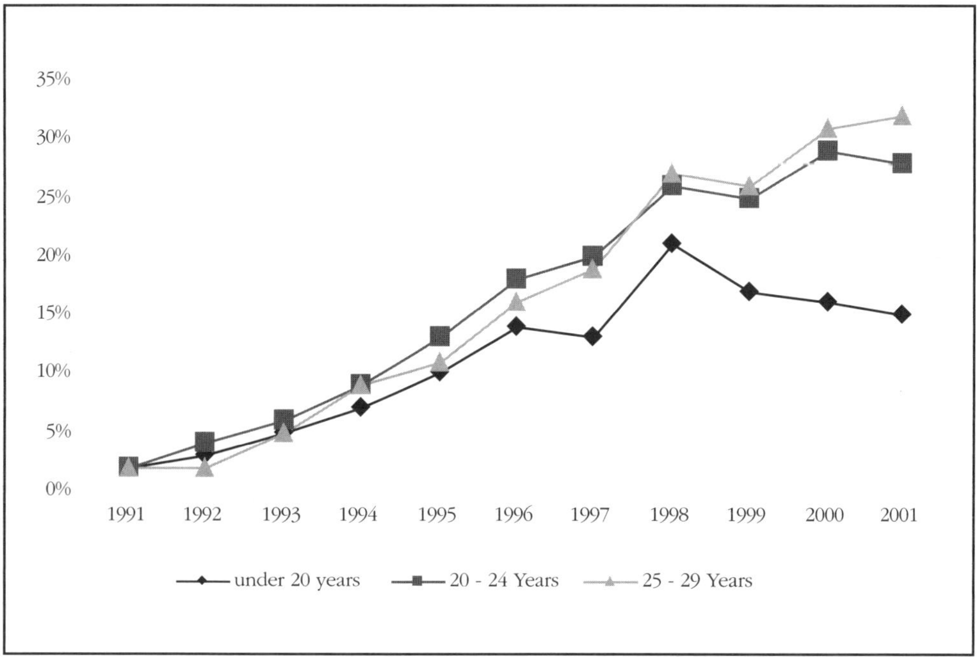

Table 2: Population pyramid in mid-2010 showing the impact of HIV/Aids on the total population[22]

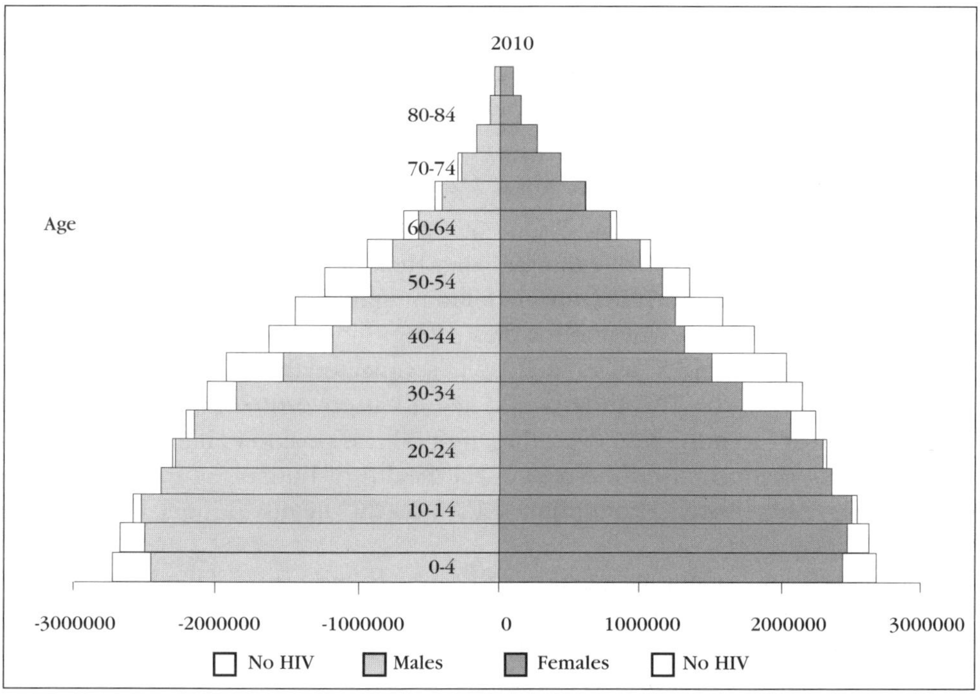

Responses to HIV and Aids in South Africa: The political context

The South African political response to HIV and Aids has been characterised by inconsistencies, absurdities and good practice. Ironically, the denial that has marked this approach was summed up in 1998 by the then Deputy President Thabo Mbeki (the man who himself was to become the centre of some of the controversies):

> *For too long we have closed our eyes as a nation, hoping the truth was not so real. At times we did not know that we were burying people who had died of Aids. At other times we knew, but chose to remain silent.*[23]

Many argue that both the apartheid and post-apartheid governments failed to respond to HIV and Aids effectively. The apartheid government failed to act due to a lack of political commitment, whilst the post-1994 government was simply overwhelmed with restructuring and developing new policies and programmes. Hence, under President Mandela's leadership – the first five years of the constitutional democracy – the HIV and Aids programme, although identified as a presidential lead project, did not effectively deal with the epidemic. Under President Mbeki – the second and current phase of the constitutional democracy – the government's stance on HIV and Aids has swung from denials to a grudging and slow acceptance of the need to follow international best practice. This position has attracted widespread criticism, particularly from the mainstream media.

There has been further criticism of Mbeki's stance on HIV and Aids since he referred to the epidemic only in passing in his state of the nation address on the 14 February 2003.[24] This resulted in attacks by the leader of the opposition in the national legislature:

> *Our response to the HIV/Aids tragedy has been one long denial. Hundreds of thousands of South Africans are dying of Aids every year, one million by the end of 2003. But we are not defenceless. Only one thing holds us back: a paralysing lack of political courage.*[25]

The confusion around the government's policy on HIV and Aids hampered programmes at all levels. For example, the Treatment Action Campaign (TAC) reported that they were unable to provide training in all of the hospitals they had targeted on the use of Nevirapine for preventing transmission of HIV from pregnant women to their babies, as some hospitals indicated that they were afraid that if they worked with the TAC they would lose their government funding.[26]

It is significant to note, however, that the political position taken by President Mbeki has not compromised the size of the health of budget or, indeed, allocations to HIV/Aids-related programmes. In fact, the health budget has steadily increased since 2000.

Consolidated national provincial health care expenditures totalled R31.966 billion in 2000, R33.835 billion in 2001 and R34.026 billion in 2002.[27] A study by the Aids Budget Unit of the Institute for Democracy in Africa (Idasa) indicates that, although overall health care expenditure remains consistent, real spending on provincial HIV/Aids conditional grants has increased: from R18 million in 2000, to R97.207 million in 2001, to R341.939 million in 2002.[28]

Amid much disquiet from social movements and the parliamentary opposition, in late 2003 the government announced a much-awaited, comprehensive plan for the treatment of people living with HIV and Aids, which some say will be the largest in the world. The government allocated R2.1 billion over the following three years to fight HIV/Aids. Media focus in this regard has been profound:

> *South Africa's anti-retroviral programme will be the largest public health intervention of its kind that the world has yet seen. There are now 350 000 people worldwide on anti-retrovirals (ARVs), 100 000 of those are in Brazil. The South African government's roll-out programme will see 53 000 people on ARVs in the first year of the programme, and 1.4 million people by the end of 2007.*[29]

The criticism has since shifted and is increasingly levelled at the state health sector for delaying the roll-out of ARVs.[30] There are still threats from the TAC to litigate against the government to force "an urgent resolution on the procurement policy for medicines."[31] While some experts, such as Francois Venter, Clinical Director of a Johannesburg-based reproductive health research unit, have been quoted in the media as criticising the state for "criminally" delaying the roll-out of ARVs, they have apparently also defended the state's comprehensive treatment initiative:[32]

> *In terms of the programme and guidelines, this is state-of-the-art stuff based on real African experience. Government has done its job, now we've got to make this public health programme work.*

Responses to HIV and Aids in South Africa: The community context

South African communities were largely silent on HIV and Aids during the first 15 years of the epidemic. In the pre-1992 era, the epidemic was simply not on the mainstream political agenda. However, in subsequent years, communities have become more and more mobilised around HIV and Aids issues. Levels of openness are increasing and more and more people wish to contribute to the fight against the epidemic; however, this is not being harnessed by the government or national institutions such as the South African National Aids Council (Sanac).

3 Institutional responses to HIV/Aids

International best practice

Good governance principles are increasingly being used as universal standards to evaluate responses to HIV and Aids. Governance is broadly defined as "a set of values, policies and institutions by which society manages its economic, political and social processes at all levels through interaction among government, civil society and private sector."[33]

The literature shows that governance in the context of HIV and Aids is best achieved through a multi-sectoral approach. Leading examples are Uganda and Thailand, which have successfully pioneered this approach. The approach is based on an acceptance that HIV and Aids is not simply a health issue, but is a developmental problem with profound socio-economic implications. A purely health-based approach is unable to deal adequately with the problem at hand, as simply treating the physical symptoms of HIV or Aids will not reduce the incidence of the disease. The social conditions that make people vulnerable to infection must be addressed as well. Furthermore, bringing in new sectors increases resources available to deal with HIV and Aids and allows for the impact on individuals, families and communities to be appropriately managed.[34]

The International Guidelines on HIV/Aids and Human Rights[35] set the international standards for a multi-sectoral response. Guideline 1 provides:

> *States should establish an effective national framework for their response to HIV/AIDS which ensures a co-ordinated, participatory, transparent and accountable approach, integrating HIV/AIDS policy and programme responsibilities, across all branches of government.*

Multi-sectoral responses in Africa

A 2002 review of national and sector policies within the SADC region established that almost all countries had a strategic plan, particularly as this was a requirement if a country wanted to apply for funding from the Global Fund for Aids, TB and Malaria (GFATM). Furthermore, all countries within the region had adopted a multi-sectoral approach to HIV and Aids. Within this type of approach many countries had established a national Aids council and typically this was located in the president's office. However, the report noted that such councils were not flourishing. Some of the difficulties faced included:

- a limited understanding of the term multi-sectoral, with some seeing it as only an expanded response within government;[36] and
- a lack of knowledge on the most appropriate ways to co-ordinate national responses to HIV/Aids.[37]

Uganda is often cited as the leading African example of a successful multi-sectoral response. The principle of a multi-sectoral and inter-sectoral response to HIV and Aids was first integrated into Ugandan policy in 1990. This was cemented in 1992 with the establishment of the Uganda Aids Commission (UAC).[38] The UAC is a statutory body that is based in the president's office[39] and its aims are to:

- enhance HIV/Aids activities in Uganda;
- develop HIV-related policies;
- facilitate HIV/Aids planning;
- disseminate information on HIV/Aids;
- mobilise resources to fight the epidemic;
- undertake advocacy for HIV/Aids activities;
- develop linkages among partners; and
- raise awareness among all Ugandans regarding HIV/Aids.[40]

The UAC has 12 members including a full-time chairperson appointed by the president. Other members are drawn from government ministries, parliament, non-governmental organisations (NGOs), people living with Aids (PLWAs), youth and women.[41] The UAC is supported by a full-time secretariat that is headed by a director general, and has three divisions, namely:

- policy;
- research and development; and
- HIV and Aids information and documentation.

The UAC operates at both national and district levels. On a national level, it meets quarterly with both government and NGO representatives.[42] Monthly technical meetings are held between the UAC, government and NGO representatives to focus on the sectoral plan harmonisation, identification of gaps, review of progress and to prepare reports for policy-makers. In addition to this, the UAC convenes short monthly meetings with its development partners to discuss policy and resource mobilisation issues; it also has two longer consultations with them every year.

Institutional responses in South Africa

The following is a brief historical description of the various HIV and Aids institutions and strategies that have been developed in South Africa.

The National Aids Co-ordinating Committee of South Africa (Nacosa) National Aids Plan

In the apartheid era, although there were national and provincial efforts initiated to address HIV and Aids, no national institutions were created and there was no national HIV and Aids strategy.

The first coherent national Aids plan was developed by Nacosa.[43] This plan (hereinafter referred to as the Nacosa Plan) was developed outside of government through a fully consultative process between the African National Congress (ANC) – before it became the ruling party in government – the Department of Health (DoH) and a wide range of sectors from within civil society.

The Nacosa Plan recognised that South Africa's response to HIV and Aids needed to be based on the principles of inter-sectoral partnerships, and hence it referred to the responsibilities of all sectors. One of the three key goals of the Nacosa Plan was to mobilise and unify provincial, international and local resources.

The Mandela government adopted the Nacosa Plan as its national HIV and Aids strategy in July 1994 and strengthened its Directorate of HIV/Aids/STDs (sexually transmitted diseases) in the DoH to ensure that it would drive the implementation process. In addition, two institutions were created to guide the response to the epidemic. The first, comprising largely extra-governmental representatives, was the Aids Advisory Group, a body of experts set up to advise the Directorate of HIV/Aids/STDs on policy matters. This Advisory Group was disbanded in 1997 following its outspoken criticism and adoption of a number of positions that were contrary to government policy. For example, it was opposed to the DoH's proposal that Aids be notifiable[44] and of the way in which the government dealt with the Virodene scandal.[45]

The second group to be established was the Inter-departmental Committee on HIV and Aids (IDC) – a forum for government departments to interact and network around HIV and Aids in the workplace.

The 1997 National Review

In 1997 a National Review of South Africa's response to HIV and Aids showed that there was a visible lack of commitment outside of the DoH to an inter-departmental approach to HIV and Aids. Although the institutional mechanisms to harness political commitment were in place, they had been ineffective. There were also criticisms of the slow implementation of the Nacosa Plan including that, at an institutional level, the implementation focused too narrowly on the health sector, particularly within the government, instead of drawing in other sectors. A further concern was that there was a lack of co-ordination between sectors and various levels, generating and/or not managing conflict between sectors.[46]

In respect of the 1997 National Review, the recommendations regarding the institutional arrangements established to respond to HIV and Aids included:

- political leadership should be secured from the Deputy President in an attempt to move the responsibility for HIV and Aids from the Ministry of Health to a person in a broader portfolio; and
- inter-departmental and inter-sectoral responses to the epidemic should be strengthened.

The 1997 Review influenced a rethinking of the institutional arrangements, and thus the Inter-ministerial Committee (IMC) on HIV and Aids was set up to facilitate the development of political commitment to addressing the epidemic. The IMC, comprising of Cabinet Ministers and their deputies, met monthly to discuss issues relating to HIV and Aids until it was disbanded at the end of 1999. It was ironically first headed by the then Deputy President Mbeki with his misguided and controversial views on HIV and Aids. The IMC was later replaced by Sanac.

The HIV/Aids Strategic Plan for South Africa: 2000–2005

Following the 1997 Review and other factors, the DoH recognised the need to develop a new strategic plan. This culminated in the HIV/Aids/STD Strategic Plan for South Africa (2000–2005) (hereinafter referred to as the 2000–2005 Strategic Plan), which is a broad strategic plan designed to guide South Africa's response to the epidemic from both within and outside government. Its stated purpose is to be a guide that can be used by every sector to develop their own strategic and operational plans, thus enabling the country to develop a harmonised, efficient and effective response to HIV and Aids.

The 2000–2005 Strategic Plan was initiated at a meeting in July 1999 where participants reviewed the existing HIV and Aids prevention, treatment and care efforts. That meeting was attended by representatives of faith-based organisations, PLWAs, human rights organisations, academic institutions, the civil-military alliance, the media, organised labour, organised sports, organised business, insurance companies, woman's organisations, youth organisations, international donor organisations, health professionals and health consulting organisations, political parties and relevant government departments.

After priority areas for future efforts were discussed and agreed upon, a committee was appointed and charged with the development of a five-year HIV/Aids/STD Strategic Plan. Task teams were established to review existing goals and objectives for the designated priority areas. The identified priority areas, around which the task teams were constituted, included prevention; treatment, care and support; legal and human rights; and monitoring, research and evaluation. In addition, the Minister of Health held bilateral meetings with several important sectors including traditional leaders, faith-based organisations and the private sector to obtain their views and to discuss ways to facilitate their active participation.

In September 1999, the Minister of Health and the nine provincial Members of the Executive Councils (MECs) for Health reconfirmed the priority areas. This was followed in October 1999 by a two-day National Aids Meeting where Provincial

Aids Co-ordinators, the National DoH, Directorate of HIV/Aids/STDs, representatives of the Aids Training and Information Centres (ATICs) and representatives of several other organisations discussed progress of the development of the five-year Strategic Plan.

In October and November 1999 the task teams met to further develop their goals and objectives. They were expected to review the Nacosa Plan, the DoH *White Paper for the Transformation of the Health System in South Africa*, the 1997 HIV/Aids/STD Review and reports from the September meeting of the Provincial MECs for Health, and the National Aids Meeting.

In November 1999 a draft document was presented to the IMC and additional comments were solicited from all government ministers. The final document, the 2000–2005 Strategic Plan, was completed in January 2000.

One of the guiding principles underlying the 2000–2005 Strategic Plan is that "all sectors of government and other stakeholders in civil society shall be involved in the fight against HIV/AIDS". Its primary goals are to reduce both the number of new infections (especially among the youth) and also the impact of HIV and Aids on individuals, families and communities. Further, the two most important bodies tasked with guiding the implementation are Sanac and the IDC.

Sanac

The government argues that it is fully supportive of an inter-sectoral approach, and the Deputy President and Chair of Sanac has publicly stated that Sanac is the embodiment of this commitment to partnerships with other sectors.[47] Furthermore, Sanac had to replace the Aids Advisory Group, as it was not a multi-sectoral body and only made up of technical experts.

The 2000–2005 Strategic Plan describes the role of Sanac as:

- advising the government on HIV and Aids policy;
- advocating for the effective involvement of sectors and organisations in implementing programmes and strategies;
- monitoring the implementation of the Strategic Plan in all sectors of society;
- creating and strengthening partnerships for an expanded response amongst all sectors;
- mobilising resources for the implementation of Aids programmes; and
- recommending appropriate research.

It was envisaged that Sanac would meet on a monthly basis; however, this issue was reviewed during October 2002 and members agreed that in future meetings would be held quarterly. In the intervening periods, the Sanac executive would meet to implement decisions and to respond to urgent matters.[48]

The 2000–2005 Strategic Plan provides that Sanac is to be made up of 34 people, 16 of whom will be from government and 17 from various sectors of civil society. It further provides that Sanac should be chaired by the Deputy President.

The government representatives should be drawn from the ministries of health; education; welfare and population development; agriculture; arts, culture, science and technology; transport; labour; finance; provincial and local government; defence; minerals and energy; correctional services; public service and administration; the deputy CEO of government communication and information systems; the chairperson of the Portfolio Committee on Health and the chairperson of the Select Committee on Social Services.

The civil society sectors that may each send one representative to Sanac include business; NGOs; faith-based organisations; trade unions; women; youth; traditional leaders; traditional healers; legal and human rights bodies; disabled people; celebrities; sport; media; hospitality industry; the National Association of People Living With HIV and Aids (NAPWA); and local government.

Nominations to Sanac were made through a public process where they were forwarded to the Directorate of HIV/Aids/STDs. The Directorate then developed a short-list, which was submitted to the President for his final decision.[49] Members are appointed for a two-year period.

Recently, Sanac has issued a call for sectors to nominate two representatives to sit on the council. In particular, they have called for nominations from businesses, organisations supporting children and orphans, academics and the "men's sector".[50]

Provincial Aids Councils (PACs)

The 2000–2005 Strategic Plan states that that each province should have its own PAC and the Cabinet endorsed this recommendation. As their mandate, the PACs would co-ordinate the provincial multi-sectoral approach with a particular focus on districts, municipalities and communities.

The terms of reference for PACs are to:

- initiate, guide and develop a Provincial Aids Plan based on the 2000–2005 Strategic Plan;
- feed back province-specific issues to Sanac;
- strengthen partnership responses amongst government departments, sectors of civil society and local spheres of government;
- mobilise resources for the provincial aids plan;
- monitor the implementation of that provincial plan; and
- advise the Provincial Cabinet on matters relating to HIV and Aids.

Table 3: Functioning Provincial Aids Councils at time of writing

Province	Functioning PAC
Eastern Cape	✓
Free State	
Gauteng	✓
KwaZulu-Natal	
Limpopo	✓
Mpumalanga	
North West	
Northern Cape	
Western Cape	✓

Membership of PACs would be similar to that of Sanac, with ministerial and sector representatives. Public nominations would be solicited and the final decision would be made by the Provincial Cabinet on the advice of the MEC for Health. The provincial Departments of Health would act as the secretariat to the PAC.

The IDC

As mentioned above, the IDC is a forum of public servants who are mandated by their departments to co-ordinate their respective departmental HIV and Aids programmes.[51] They are mandated to:

- develop workplace HIV and Aids programmes and policies; and
- ensure government departments allocate resources to HIV and Aids.

The IDC has a plenary body made up of representatives from each national government department. The two co-chairs, who are elected for a one-year period by the ordinary members, and a full-time secretariat, based in the DoH to support the IDC, form a steering committee for more effective management. A number of ad hoc task teams, which undertake specific functions, provide additional support to the IDC.[52] There are no plans at present to move the secretariat of the IDC from the DoH as it is currently the department with the most capacity to manage the programme.

The IDC works with a number of structures within government, including Sanac, the Directors General Social Cluster (an inter-departmental co-ordination structure comprising Directors General dealing with social matters), provincial IDCs, the Department of Public Administration's Impact and Acton Project, the DoH's Government Aids Action Plan and its Partnership Support Programme.[53]

An annual participatory planning workshop, convened by the IDC, determines the activities for the year and elects the new co-chairs.[54] All decisions are taken by the plenary or the steering committee. Generally, proposals are put forward by task teams or members and are ratified at the IDC meeting.[55] The agenda is set by the steering committee. Minutes are kept of all meetings. Although this has not been confirmed, it appears that the minutes are public documents and could be requested through the secretariat.[56]

Funding for the IDC is provided by the DoH from its European Union funds. The DoH must approve all expenditure and account for funds spent. It currently has a budget of less than R1 million. Of these funds, roughly 40 per cent is spent on the staffing and operational costs of the secretariat, and 60 per cent is spent on operations. IDC members are not paid for the time they spend on IDC work.[57]

In its work the IDC has in the past focused primarily on workplace HIV and Aids programmes; however, at a recent planning event it was agreed that there was a need to widen this focus and provide support to other departmental HIV/Aids activities.[58]

Reports are written every four months and submitted to the Directors General Social Cluster. The IDC submits an annual written report to Sanac, an annual verbal report to the abovementioned Social Cluster and, as the secretariat is based in the DoH, a report to the Chief Director of HIV/Aids/STDs.[59]

The secretariat of the IDC reports that it has a culture of being independent and making decisions on the basis of consensus. However, members of the IDC often struggle with the fact that departmental line managers, to whom they are accountable, undervalue this work and the time given to the IDC.[60]

The IDC secretariat has identified a number of problems the IDC has faced in carrying out its mandate. These include:

- insufficient links between the IDC and the Directors General Social Cluster;
- the junior position of most IDC members;
- lack of communication between IDC members and their senior management;
- insufficient resources allocated to HIV and Aids programmes within departments; and
- insufficient project management and monitoring in many departments.[61]

An external evaluation of the IDC is planned during 2004.[62]

There are 37 national government departments (including standing commissions). In practice, the IDC reports, roughly 27 departments are represented and participate in one way or another on the IDC. Furthermore, the IDC secretariat reports that approximately 33.3 per cent of IDC members are actively involved in its work. The IDC has not formally examined its composition but it reports that it is racially representative and more women and then men participate in its work. Regarding the skills of members of the IDC, it was reported that "IDC members tend to be reasonably skilled in HIV and Aids matters and the workplace programmes. Due to a high turnover in staff, skills building is an ongoing need. Generally there is a lack in programme management skills."[63]

Other institutions

There are other institutional structures that also take decisions relating to HIV and Aids. They include:

- the Cabinet;
- MinMec (a forum in which the MECs of health meet with the national minister to discuss issues of common concern); and
- the Directors General Forum (a forum of Directors General within all government departments who meet to discuss issues of common concern across the public service).

4 Institutional appraisal of South Africa's HIV and Aids response

Summary of criteria used

An institutional appraisal is an assessment of the external and internal factors affecting organisational performance and outputs. Good governance principles indicate that the most appropriate manner to respond to HIV and Aids is by way of a multi-sectoral, multi-dimensional programme. In this appraisal we have reviewed Sanac by examining its:

- structure;
- organisational culture;
- management systems and processes; and
- people.

It should be noted that this institutional appraisal was a study of the perceptions of various role-players on the effectiveness of Sanac in promoting a multi-sectoral response to HIV/Aids in South Africa. This was not an official evaluation of Sanac.

Structure

The structure of an organisation is important as this:

- facilitates decision-making;
- clarifies roles and responsibilities;
- organises resources; and
- influences organisational culture.

In this instance, the factors we have used to determine whether Sanac is an effective institution are:

- the nature of its structure and whether it facilitates the members meeting their mandate;
- the extent to which it is representative, and especially whether vulnerable groups are represented or are able to participate in its work;
- the ability of non-members to participate in proceedings (whether mecha-

nisms exist to allow for such participation), and linked to this the extent to which Sanac is accessible to members of civil society;
- the extent to which Sanac has interacted with other stakeholders such as international donor agencies; and
- whether Sanac is accountable to the public.

Organisational culture

Good governance literature indicates that for an inter-sectoral response to be successful, it must be supported by political commitment and an organisational environment that promotes healthy, collaborative relationships between government, civil society and the private sector.[64] Decisions must be openly discussed and effectively communicated to all citizens, and processes must be developed to allow citizens to participate in decision-making.[65] In accordance with the theoretical models of institutional culture, we will examine the power, roles, tasks and people in assessing the organisational culture of Sanac.

The specific criteria that have been used include:
- whether Sanac systems and organisational culture are based on democratic values;
- the extent to which Sanac is free from political interference and is able to act independently; and
- whether the management style within Sanac encourages participation and inclusiveness in decision-making.

Systems and processes

An institution cannot be effective unless it has appropriate management systems and processes that meet the needs of its target groups.

> *Good governance ensures that political, social and economic priorities are based on broad consensus in society and that the voices of the poorest of the poor and the most vulnerable are heard in decision-making and the allocation of resources.*[66]

The specific criteria that have been used include whether Sanac has:
- planning processes and strategic plans in place;
- financial management systems to ensure proper accounting of all public and donor funds;
- systems that facilitate effective and productive work;
- regular reviews and evaluations;
- outputs that meet the goals set for the institutions.

People

People form the final but crucial element of an institution. Without the appropriate skills and diversity within the institution, it will be unable to meet its objectives.

The specific criteria used include:

- appropriateness of the size of the institution and its constituent bodies;
- members being representative of relevant groups including vulnerable groups;
- members having appropriate skills and knowledge; and
- members displaying leadership to others.

Structure

Description

Sanac has a simple organisational structure. It has an executive, a plenary body, advisory technical task teams and a secretariat.

Table 4: Structure of Sanac

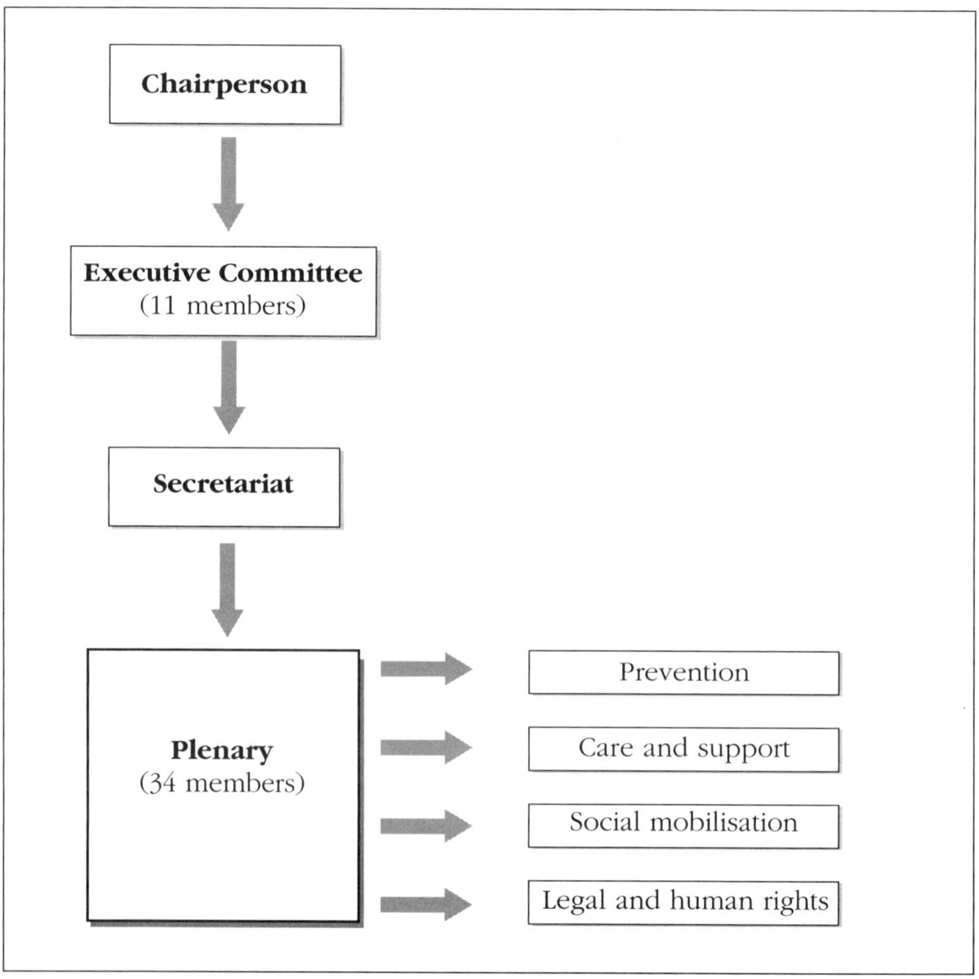

This structure has been adopted to facilitate the achievement of a number of core functions, including what has been described as its primary role:

> *At the time of the establishment of Sanac, discourse on HIV/Aids in the country was focused on government's apparent inability to deal effectively with the epidemic. The media was hostile and the DoH was under constant criticism. Against this background, Sanac was established as an attempt to get civil society on board and create the foundation for an inclusive structure.*[67]

Other functions include:

- advising government on policy development;
- advocacy for the greater involvement of all sectors;
- monitoring and evaluation;
- developing and enhancing partnerships;
- mobilising resources; and
- recommending appropriate research.[68]

Within this general framework, each of the constituent elements of Sanac has specific functions.

Executive

The executive is mandated to deal with urgent matters and oversee the implementation of programmes. It is envisaged that it will meet on a regular (monthly or fortnightly) basis.[69] It has also been reported that it will attempt to develop closer links with the PACs.[70] The executive is made up of nine members: five Cabinet Ministers, a member of Napwa, a representative from the women's sector, the hospitality sector and Cosatu[71] (see Appendix 4 for a list of members of the executive).

Plenary

The heart of Sanac is its plenary, which is made up of 33 members, the various sectoral representatives, and is chaired by the Deputy President (see Appendix 3 for a list of its current members).

Technical task teams

The plenary is advised by five technical task teams, which are made up of experts in the following areas:

- prevention;
- care and support;
- information, education and communication and social mobilisation;
- research, monitoring, surveillance and evaluation; and
- legal issues and human rights.

Secretariat

Sanac is supported in its work by a three-person secretariat, which was based, for Sanac's first term of office, in the DoH's Directorate of HIV/Aids/STDs. In March 2003 the Sanac secretariat moved out of the DoH to its own offices. Its functions include:

- collecting background information for meetings;
- drafting analytical reports and position papers;
- undertaking all logistical support for Sanac meetings; and
- recording and distributing the minutes of all meetings.[72]

Sanac currently has no other dedicated staff besides its secretariat. However, in an internal Sanac document, it is proposed that five additional staff members be appointed:

- a project manager, at the level of deputy director, to oversee the work of the secretariat;
- a senior state accountant, at the level of assistant or deputy director, to ensure efficient financial management of Sanac funds;
- a communications expert to deal with all Sanac communications; and
- two administrators to support the secretariat.[73]

The appointment of staff, as articulated in the framework document, will be pursued by contracting a consultant who will assist Sanac in developing terms of reference and the staffing structure it requires to meet its mandate.[74]

Criticism of the Sanac structure

Sanac's structure has been criticised by a number of NGOs.

- The Aids Consortium argues that Sanac's current structure does not allow it to be transparent and representative. They would like to see Sanac restructured into a Country Co-ordinating Mechanism (CCM) as envisaged by the GFATM. The TAC agrees with the Aids Consortium's views.[75]
- There is no full-time paid staff and thus Sanac's ability to take on substantive issues is compromised. For example, the TAC sees this as a major structural flaw. They state that one of the primary roles of Sanac should be to lead the development of a national treatment plan. However, they argue that in its current form, Sanac is unable to undertake such a task.[76] The TAC has stated that Sanac should:

  > *...develop and facilitate the implementation of a national treatment plan, besides antiretroviral therapy. Part of this plan must be the implementation of antiretroviral community treatment programmes in urban and rural health facilities in every province within the next six months. Other essential components of, or closely related to, a treatment plan include voluntary counselling and testing, mother to child transmission prevention of HIV/Aids, better*

management of STDs, post exposure prophylaxis for rape survivors, substantial increases in public health-funding, unfreezing of essential health care posts and poverty relief measures, such as the Basic Income Grant.[77]

- The current structure has allowed the DoH to continue to dominate Sanac. The secretariat was placed within the DoH and they effectively set the agenda for all meetings; this meant that other sectors were not given an equal opportunity to place issues on the Sanac agenda.[78] The DoH was thus not transparent in its approach to setting the agenda.

The lack of a structural mechanism to interface particularly with NGOs appears to be a common criticism of Sanac.[79] Sanac is not accountable to anyone; it does not report to any structure and its minutes and proceedings are kept confidential.[80]

SANAC has never managed to profile itself as the leading HIV and Aids body in South Africa. This is in contrast to the high esteem in which the Uganda Aids Commission is held. For example, a commentator in a paper on HIV and governance noted:

> *Sanac has been largely conspicuous by its absence so far. Its public profile is limited, which is disappointing given the axiomatic role it is intended to play, and it has not yet leapt into action, though it meets once a month …*[81]

In an interview with Mark Heywood, the head of the Aids Law Project, he remarked that Sanac had been marginalised by the fact that, despite various controversies around HIV such as the appointment of a Presidential Panel on HIV/Aids and the Nevirapine constitutional court case,[82] there had never been consultations by government with other sectors represented in Sanac on any of these issues.[83]

Recommendations for restructuring Sanac

Two proposals have been made for the restructuring of Sanac, one by the Aids Consortium and the TAC and the other by Dr J Sachs, a consultant employed by Sanac.

The Aids Consortium and the TAC recommended that Sanac be reconstituted in the form of a CCM. A CCM is a broad-based partnership within a country. It should be made up of government ministries, NGOs/CBOs, people living with HIV or Aids, private sector companies, international NGOs and agencies, and bi- and multi-lateral agencies. Such a body should have a mandate to:

> *...work together to develop a multi-sectoral plan for fighting Aids, TB and Malaria. Furthermore the stakeholders would be, in most instances, participating in the implementation of the activities as well as monitoring and evaluation.*[84]

This means that for Sanac to bring itself into line with the GFATM's requirements, it should ensure that the private sector and international agencies and NGOs are more fullly represented. It would also have to strengthen its ability to implement, monitor and evaluate programmes.

Dr Sachs recommended restructuring Sanac into an executive body that could be accountable to the Cabinet. This body should interface with the different sectors, technical task teams and communities. In order to strengthen the HIV and Aids response within government, HIV and Aids directorates should be established in additional ministries such as education.[85]

An appraisal of the Sanac structure

Does Sanac's structure enable it to meet its mandate?

In theory, the Sanac structure is sound. It is essentially a plenary body that represents a number of different sectors, giving them all an opportunity to meet, interact and network on HIV and Aids issues. However, in practice, its structure has been a major obstacle to it fulfilling its mandate for a number of different reasons.

Firstly, Sanac's structure is dominated by government representatives (49 per cent of its members represent the state in some form). Eighty per cent of the government representatives are Cabinet Ministers, and the others include parliamentary and government communication representatives. By allowing Sanac's structure to be dominated by government representatives, it has:

- created an impression that Sanac is not an independent body;
- indicated that the government regards itself as the most important sector in the response to the epidemic; and
- taken responsibility away from other sectors.[86]

This research project was not able to establish why the government needed so many representatives on the Council. It seems particularly unnecessary to have so many Cabinet Ministers on both the plenary and executive, as they seldom attend meetings and are generally too busy to take on additional Sanac work.

Secondly, although nothing in this structure prevents it from advising government on policy development, this has not happened.[87] The framework document states that this was "not by design but by default" and is largely because all government departments have clearly laid out policy development procedures that do not involve consulting Sanac.

Thirdly, its structure does not allow it to monitor the implementation of the 2000–2005 Strategic Plan within either the government or civil society. It is unable to effectively monitor the work of the government, as it is not structurally independent from the government. It is also difficult to monitor implementation within the private sector, as no clear indicators have been set for what each sector should achieve.

Fourthly, its structure does not allow it to interact with other stakeholders or any non-members, except through the sectoral representatives. Unlike the Uganda Aids Commission, it does not have consultations with NGOs or other sectors.

Fifthly, its structure has not enabled it to form strategic partnerships with other organisations, donors or sectors excluded from Sanac, as it does not have any mechanism for interacting with these groups. The only way it interacts with others is through the work of each of its sectoral representatives.

Does the Sanac structure ensure that it represents key stakeholders and vulnerable groups?

Vulnerable groups are represented on Sanac. Fifteen percent of its members represent women, youth and the disabled (see Tables 5 and 6, pps 39–40). People living with HIV or Aids are also represented in the plenary and the executive. A notable group that is excluded is organisations working with children. It has been reported that this sector was to be represented on Sanac from 1 April 2003, when the new Sanac will have been constituted.[88]

Does the Sanac structure facilitate the participation of non-members?

It appears that the Sanac structure does not facilitate the participation of non-members. The private sector, donors, organisations, NGOs and CBOs can only engage with Sanac through their sectoral representative, if they have one. There is no other structural mechanism for allowing such groups to influence the agenda of meetings or the work of Sanac.

Furthermore, Sanac does appear not to be accountable to non-members or other sectors, as its meetings are closed, minutes are not available and it does not make any reports public.

Sanac's inability to interact with civil society is a key limitation on its ability to fulfil its mandate.

Case Study: Failure of Sanac to interact with stakeholders

The Aids Consortium has tried to get Sanac to discuss a national treatment plan and even offered to present on this issue; however, it has never received any feedback on this issue and are aware that the subject has never been placed on the agenda.[89]

The TAC has tried to get Sanac to discuss the treatment plan which was tabled for discussion at Nedlac; however, it was told that Sanac was not an "appropriate forum" for such a discussion. An offer was made to present the draft treatment plan to Sanac but no response was received.[90]

Does the Sanac structure enable it to be accountable to the public?
There is no structural impediment to Sanac being accountable to the public. Most of the problems with accountability lie in its internal systems and processes. The only significant structural problem is that it does not report to any public body such as parliament.

Does the Sanac structure create mechanisms to make it accessible to the public?
It appears that the current structure does not in any way make the body accessible to the public. There is no mechanism for the public to write to, send submissions to or even request a hearing before Sanac. In the framework document, Sanac refers to the fact that it has held meetings outside of Pretoria; however, as these meetings were closed to the public, their venue in no way enhanced their accessibility.

Organisational culture

Description

The organisational culture of Sanac has been approached by examining its values, its independence, the participation of its members and political commitment to its work.

Organisational values
Sanac does not have any internal policy documents that set out guidelines for participation, but the respondents who were involved in Sanac agreed that there was some form of participation by sectors, and decisions were made on the basis of consensus.[91]

Independence
Sanac is not a statutory body. In its first term of office it was essentially "managed" by the DoH, as it provided all the technical support and finances for Sanac's activities. For Sanac's second term of office a trust fund has been set up and all its finances will be managed by the trustees.[92] Its secretariat has also moved out of the DoH to its own offices outside of any government department.

Participation
Sanac members can participate by being part of the executive, attending plenary meetings, interacting with the technical task teams and facilitating the greater involvement of their sector in the implementation of the 2000–2005 Strategic Plan.

There is currently no interaction between Sanac and non-members; all interactions with the general public take place through the sectoral representatives. There is, however, a press statement released after every meeting to keep the public informed on new developments.[93]

Political commitment
SANAC is chaired by the Deputy President Jacob Zuma, and 12 of his fellow Cabinet Ministers are members of the Council. The presence of so many political leaders on Sanac provides it with political credibility and an ability to influence decision-making at the highest level – this is particularly important given the fact that the Cabinet is also a major role-player in the co-ordination and implementation of the HIV and Aids strategies.

Criticisms of Sanac's organisational culture

A number of individuals and NGOs have criticised Sanac's organisational culture. A common concern regarding the values of Sanac is its real or perceived lack of independence. The Aids Consortium, for example, has argued that this has led to Sanac only responding to issues that were not in conflict with current government policy. In an interview it put this quite bluntly:

> *Sanac have never taken a single independent stand on issues...they have huge problems relating to independence. Problems are due to their ties to government through funding and their government-based secretariat.*[94]

The Aids Consortium argues that this "tainted" image of Sanac will be difficult to shrug off even if it is restructured.

Recommendations for the reform of Sanac

Organisational Culture
Only one recommendation was made for the development of a better organisational culture within Sanac. The women's sector representative on Sanac argued that the best way to improve the independence of Sanac was through its sectoral representatives. If they brought independent voices to Sanac this would help to ensure that the body was not a rubber stamp for government policies.

An appraisal of Sanac's institutional culture

Does Sanac have a culture of democracy?
At face value it appears that sectors participate within Sanac and there is a culture of decisions based only on consensus.[95] It was noted with concern that there was an unofficial sense that it would be inappropriate to criticise government policy within Sanac.[96] Thus, participation takes place within this culture of silence and acquiescence.

Is Sanac independent?
There are two issues regarding the independence of Sanac, namely its independence from the government generally and its independence from the DoH.

Regarding the first issue, this is a complex problem. It appears that any body that is chaired by the Deputy President cannot be independent from the government. Such a body would not be in a position to strongly condemn the government's position on a particular policy or programme. This means that the process within Sanac could be independent; even in a body that is chaired by the Deputy President members should feel confident to voice their opinions, whether supportive or critical of government policy.

There appears to be a tension between political commitment, as manifested by representation by government officials and politicians, and real independence. Having Sanac chaired by the Deputy President certainly brings with it political commitment at the highest level. In a South African context it seems that this tension between political commitment via representation and independence has resulted in a double loss to Sanac. Not only has it impaired the perception of Sanac as an independent body but the Ministers have failed to use their political commitment, and as a result most departments have not moved forward significantly in terms of HIV policy and planning since 2000.

Regarding the second issue, it appears that this is a problem of the DoH trying to assert some control over Sanac. It has been reported that there have been clashes between the Minister of Health, with her unorthodox views on HIV, and the Chairperson of Sanac, Deputy President Zuma, who takes a more mainstream view on HIV.[97] This tension between denialists and mainstreamers apparently ripples right through Sanac with the existence of two clear camps.[98] It makes the work of Sanac particularly difficult, as it has been so dependant on the DoH for capacity and resources.

However, real steps have been taken to address this issue; the secretariat has been moved out of the DoH, its finances are now being managed by an independent trust fund and steps are being taken to employ staff. All these steps will help to reduce Sanac's reliance on the DoH's Directorate of HIV/Aids/STDs.

Does the management style within Sanac encourage participation?

It is not clear whether the management style within Sanac encourages participation. A number of respondents reported that participation was good. However, others argued that Sanac did not encourage participation of all sectors. Apparently, Sanac meetings are dominated by government representatives who spend hours reporting on their programmes and justifying state policies.[99] Sanac itself seems to recognise this, as informal reports indicate that it is aware that the focus of meetings has been on the government's HIV and Aids programmes and not on developing policy or on getting sectoral reports.[100]

Decision-making within Sanac was described as follows:

> *No major decisions are made...because Sanac is government dominated, civil society is not heard...usually decisions are deferred to the DoH who then just give an explanation to Sanac members.*[101]

Sanac's inability to create an open and accepting environment for different views is also illustrated by its approach to setting the agenda. It was reported to an Aids Consortium meeting that the agendas for Sanac meetings were always predetermined and sectors could not make an input into this process.[102] Furthermore, the agenda is only available on the day of the meeting, which prevents the sector representatives from obtaining mandates or even consulting their constituencies on the issues being discussed.[103]

The TAC describes the problem as follows:

> *Regrettably, Sanac civil society members have not been able to actively influence the agenda of this body and have remained prisoner to the agenda of the government.*[104]

Is there political commitment towards Sanac's work?

Although Sanac has the potential to harness political commitment in favour of HIV and Aids, it appears to be a political body that is sidelined at every level when it comes to key decisions on HIV and Aids. Illustrating this point, a respondent referred to the Cabinet decision on 17 April 2002 to support the development of a national treatment plan. Sanac was not consulted on this issue and has not acted on it:

> *The 17 April 2002 statement by Cabinet has never led to any implementation by Sanac. They should have had a meeting regarding this issue to see how the various sectors could respond and implement treatment plans.*[105]

Two key problems emerge regarding political commitment; firstly, Sanac's inability to be part of key processes regarding HIV and Aids decision-making and, secondly, its inability to make an impact on the outcome of key decisions which are being made. Therefore, it is not bringing political commitment to the HIV and Aids response in South Africa.

Case study: The GFAMT and the Enhancing Care Initiative (ECI) dispute with Sanac

> *In its first round of funding, the GFAMT approved 29 of the 332 proposals it had received, with 10 per cent of the funds they approved, earmarked for South Africa.*[106]

The GFAMT received 15 proposals from South Africa; however, they elected to fund only two – one submitted by Sanac for US$91 million and the proposal from the ECI[107] for an amount of US$72 million.

One of the funding requirements was that the proposal be submitted by a CCM, broadly defined as a body representing a wide range of stakeholders who would co-ordinate the programme. The GFATM provided that the CCM may be a state or civil society structure. Both successful South African proposals were submitted by bodies considering themselves to be CCMs.

However, following the notification that their proposal was successful, the ECI was informed by Sanac that there were procedural irregularities with their proposal as it had not been submitted through the "official" CCM and, as a result of this, the DoH indicated that it would re-divide the grant amongst all nine provinces – a proposal which placed the funding in jeopardy. This resulted in a protracted dispute between the ECI, Sanac, the DoH and the GFATM.

This dispute is a useful case study as it reflects many of the broader problems with Sanac.

Sanac's real and perceived lack of independence

Press reports indicate a perception of political interference in donor funding applications. The ECI considers this too simplistic an analysis. In fact, it argues that proposals based on extending access to ARVs within the public health system are more likely to face political obstructionism due to the underlying political commitment to Aids denial.

The difficult boundaries between the DoH and Sanac

The DoH acted as the "official" spokesperson for Sanac in this dispute, thus again showing that Sanac is not truly independent of the DoH.

Government control over Sanac processes

The Sanac proposal was prepared by the DoH with little consultation of the civil society sector and without the knowledge even of many Sanac members.[108] This appears to be part of a broader problem relating to unwillingness to share the management of donor funds with a range of stakeholders as is required by the GFATM.

An inability to deal with conflict and problems

This problem becomes particularly acute when the issues are raised in the media. The University of Natal (the home of ECI) is reported as saying that no one within Sanac was prepared to take responsibility and deal with the dispute.[109] Thus, unless the organisational culture within Sanac changes, this type of problem will persist, as there is a fundamental lack of trust and clear communication between Sanac and other stakeholders.

In conclusion, the Minister of Health for KwaZulu-Natal, Dr Zweli Mkhize, later reported to the provincial parliament that amendments had been made to the ECI proposal to the GFATM to bring it in line with national and provincial strategies on HIV and Aids. He further stated that despite the amendments, the proposal "still has all the essential elements it had – what has happened is that the proposal has been refined".[110]

Systems and processes

Description

Obtaining information on Sanac's systems and process was difficult, as no formal policy documents were available.

Planning
Sanac has an annual planning meeting; however, it does not have a strategic plan setting out its objectives against a budget.[111] For its first term of office, the final planning session was held in October 2002. In terms of a broader framework, it works within the strategic objectives set out in the 2000–2005 Strategic Plan.

Management systems
In its first term of office all management functions were provided by the DoH. In other words, all finances were allocated and accounted for in accordance with the department's own rules and regulations. Secretariat support was also provided by DoH staff. In its second term of office Sanac will be managing its own funds and staff. It could not be established whether any management polices of procedures had been developed or whether the systems used within the DoH would also be used within the newly "independent" Sanac.

Reviews
Sanac has no formal policy on how it should monitor, evaluate and review its work. It appears that sectors do report on their work at Sanac meetings, although how regularly this takes place could not be established.

In the second half of Sanac's first term of office it conducted an internal review of its work[112] and this was followed by the appointment of an external evaluator, Dr Sachs, in October 2002 who undertook a "review of the two years of existence of Sanac and related bodies with the aim of provoking discussion on necessary structural adjustments".[113]

Outputs
The objectives of Sanac are set out in the DoH's five-year Strategic Plan.

Sanac is not a statutory body and participation in it is voluntary and without remuneration. It was argued that this has had a significant impact on its outputs.[114] Furthermore, all the members are in full-time employment and are extremely busy. This makes devoting time to Sanac difficult and it also impacts on meeting attendance. The extent to which Sanac has been able to achieve its objectives will be discussed below.

Criticisms of Sanac's management processes and systems

Most criticisms relate to the lack of meetings. In the two years since its inception, only eight Sanac meetings have been held. It was reported to the Aids Consortium meeting on 28 October 2002 that there were only three meetings in 2002 (in February, May and October). In general, all the meetings have been irregular. Furthermore, representatives were informed at the last minute or meetings were cancelled without notice.[115] The Deputy President subsequently reported that although not many meetings were held in 2002, two meetings had already been held in 2003, the first on the 21 January (executive committee) and the second on 1 February (full council).[116]

The lack of meetings leads to the problem of the agenda being overloaded as issues pile up.[117] This creates difficulty in dealing with critical issues extensively and makes it difficult for members to participate effectively.

A further problem with meetings is that although Cabinet Ministers make up 36 per cent of Sanac members, it appears that they seldom attend meetings. Members of the civil society sector of Sanac seem to have attended meetings more regularly, although there are some notable exceptions. This is a difficult issue to address as all Sanac members are highly committed to their full-time jobs and other activities. Cabinet Ministers in particular have full diaries, which are planned months in advance, making the setting of meetings extremely difficult.

An appraisal of Sanac's systems and processes

Does Sanac have a strategic plan and an annual planning process?

There appear to be two parallel planning processes that need to take place within Sanac – its own planning and the planning for the work within each sector. Both seem to be in place to some extent, although there are some problems:

- despite its planning process, Sanac does not have an operational nor medium- or long-term plan;
- the various sectors seem to be at very different stages of planning;
- the focus still appears to be on sectors developing plans and applying for funding from the DoH or Sanac to support these plans.[118] This does not build sustainability or commitment within the sectors. Neither is this squarely in line with the objectives of Sanac;
- there seems to be no intention to make sector or Sanac plans public.

Does Sanac have financial systems in place to enable it to properly account for the use of its budget?

The Sanac budget has been sizeable, at R10 million for both the 2001/2002[119] and 2002/2003 financial years.[120] Whilst R15 million was allocated for the 2003/2004 financial year,[121] it was not possible to obtain confirmation on how the budget was spent. Even though Sanac members were provided with this information it was on the understanding that it was not to be made public.[122]

The DoH managed Sanac funding until the 2003/2004 budget and would have been accounted for by the Minister of Health as part of the overall health budget. However, from the next budget cycle the funding will be disbursed from a trust fund.

There are a number of unanswered questions regarding the Sanac trust fund. Many have been identified by Sanac itself, and include the following:

- who will the trustees be and how many of them will be civil society representatives?
- what financial controls will be in place to ensure that trust funds are properly accounted for?
- will the public have access to information on the trust?
- will the trust have the ability to act as a fundraiser and what legal implications does this have in terms of current legislation?
- how should government support Sanac (by diverting funds from the DoH or directly from the treasury)?
- how can the trust ensure that sectors also contribute towards its costs?

Does Sanac have systems to enhance productivity?

It appears that Sanac does not have any systems to enhance productivity. This has impacted on its accountability, transparency and its capacity to fulfil its tasks. Key problems include:

- there is no way to determine which members are productive and effective;
- there is no accountability if members do not perform;
- no-one is bound by Sanac decisions;[123]
- the secretariat is left with most tasks;
- meetings are infrequent and often cancelled at short notice;
- the agenda becomes loaded due to infrequent meetings and this prevents non-members from placing issues before Sanac. It also means that the meetings focus on routine issues and government department reports rather than policy issues.[124]

Furthermore, members who attempted to mobilise their sectors faced numerous obstacles. Work within Sanac itself was fraught with difficulties, as is illustrated by an examination of the work of the Technical Task Teams.

Case study: The technical task teams

At its inception, five technical task teams were set up to assist Sanac with its work. These task teams do not seem to be operational at present, with meetings not being held and no communication existing between the task teams and Sanac. Furthermore, it was never clear what the role and mandate of the technical task teams would be and how they would on the one hand advice Sanac and on the other work with the DoH's HIV/Aids and STDs programme. Mark Heywood, the Chairperson of the Law and Human Rights Task Team, expressed his frustration that although he did a presentation to Sanac on key human rights issues during February 2001, he never received any further feedback. As far as he is aware only one of the issues, relating to insurance, was ever taken further.[125]

The difficulties of working within Sanac appear to be as follows:

- only limited support is available from the Sanac secretariat, as it does not have full-time programme staff;
- no clear guidelines exist on when and how sectors may apply for funding to support planned activities;
- the secretariat involves itself in substantive issues relating to how sectoral funding is spent. For example, when funding was allocated to the PLWA sector to elect a new representative to Sanac, the secretariat was alleged to have made all the decisions about the summit's objectives;[126]
- there is no operational plan to guide activities;
- no clear link exists between the technical task teams and the Sanac plenary. In their reports to Sanac in October 2002, four out of five teams reported that their key challenge was their relationship with Sanac;
- there is a lack of clarity on Sanac's role.

Best practice

Elize Levendal, the Sanac women's sector representative, went out of her way to ensure that the women's sector engaged with Sanac. She worked with the DoH's HIV/Aids Partnership Support Programme and began by writing to all the women's organisations to ask their opinions on the role of Sanac. Using this information and funds supplied by the DoH, she facilitated the establishment of the Women's Partnership Against Aids.

Does Sanac have mechanisms for reviewing its work?

It appears clear that Sanac is aware of the need to review its work. An internal review of Sanac took place in October 2002; however, it did not include or allow participation by any external stakeholders. The TAC criticised this approach, asking what the purpose of a review was without considering the views of those calling for Sanac to be restructured.[127]

Media reports indicate that the October 2002 planning meeting of Sanac was supplied with a report prepared by the DoH critically reviewing Sanac's work to date. This review, although distributed to members of Sanac, does not appear to be available in the public domain. However, press statements following this review indicated that agreement had been reached on the need to improve outputs by:

- strengthening Sanac's secretariat;
- broadening NGO representation on the Council; and
- allowing sectors to nominate their own representatives.[128]

Following this, the Deputy President issued a statement on 19 February 2003 in which he has defensively asserted that:

> *Sanac is fully functional and executes its tasks effectively as required by its mandate. It is the embodiment of the country's Partnership against Aids, and is the best-qualified body to harness and process the country's multi-sectoral response to the epidemic as it represents all key sectors and constituencies.*[129]

An external evaluator, Dr Johnny Sachs also confirmed that he had undertaken an external review of Sanac during 2002, and a discussion document he prepared was made available to this research project; however, it was agreed that the outcomes of the overall review would be kept confidential.[130]

A number of changes to Sanac's structure have taken place since this review, and all have been referred to above.

Another monitoring mechanism is the sectoral reports made by representatives to Sanac. This appears to be an effective way of establishing the progress being made in different sectors.

Is Sanac meeting its objectives?

It appears that Sanac is not meeting its objectives in most areas.

Advising government on policy matters: As stated above, this has not occurred at all, largely because Sanac is not part of formal policymaking structures within government departments. Mark Heywood argues that it is also because Sanac has been sidelined from key decisions.

Mobilising civil society to become involved in the Strategic Plan: Sanac reports that in this area they were highly successful.[131] However, careful analysis of the sectoral reports show that of the 35 government sectors that were required to report 26 per cent did not submit a report.[132] The tasks undertaken by the other sectors that did report focused only on HIV prevention, with 42 per cent undertaking Aids awareness, 17 per cent training, 0.6 per cent providing counselling services and a shocking 0.02 per cent reporting any broader interaction with their sector.[133] Therefore, it cannot be argued that the government is facilitating the involvement of sectors in the Strategic Plan. Regarding reports from other sectors, 11 reports were presented; again the focus was on prevention, with 64 per cent reporting that they undertook Aids awareness activities. However, an encouraging 55 per cent reported that they undertook advocacy campaigns within their sectors.

Monitoring the implementation of the strategic plan: Sanac itself admits that this has not been done.[134]

Developing and strengthening partnerships to respond to HIV/Aids: The Council argues that this is one of its most successful areas of work. In an article in the *Aids Bulletin*,[135] Michelle Rotchford Galloway argues that this is the most important function of Sanac. She says that Sanac should be strengthening partnerships between local and international bodies and NGOs and should act as a platform for dialogue between sectors. Although this has occurred to some extent through Sanac developing new partnerships, it has not done sufficient to enhance its partnerships with local NGOs, donors and international agencies. This has been lacking, as meetings are too infrequent, not all sectors are represented and sector representatives have in the past been determined by the government and not by the sectors themselves.

Best practice

Sanac has facilitated the development of partnerships against Aids through the establishment of the Men's Forum, the Partnership with Pick 'n Pay and the Women's Partnership Against Aids.

A framework document on the restructuring of Sanac

Mobilising resources to combat HIV/Aids: Sanac admits that it has been unable to attract any additional funding over and above the funds allocated by the DoH and more recently the GFATM. It argues that the establishment of the trust fund will enable it to address this problem in the future.

Recommend appropriate research: This is an area in where Sanac has not contributed at all. It does not have representation of scientists on the Council and it has not made any efforts to engage with the Medical Research Council or other academic research institutions.

People

Description

Composition and size

Sanac is made up of 34 members, 16 representing sectors within government (13 of whom are Cabinet Ministers) and 17 representing civil society sectors. They were all appointed for a two-year term from December 1999–2001. The term was extended to March 2003 by the Deputy President.[136]

Representation

The sectors represented within Sanac include:

- government (Cabinet Ministers and the government communication and information services);
- parliament;
- business;
- PLWAs;
- NGOs;
- faith-based organisations;
- trade unions;
- women;
- youth;
- traditional leaders;
- legal and human rights groups;
- disabled people;
- celebrities;
- sporting bodies;
- local government; and
- the hospitality industry.

Capacity

Not all the persons represented on Sanac are HIV/Aids experts or come from HIV/Aids organisations. Capacity varies.

Criticisms of the composition and people within Sanac

From its inception, Aids activists and experts criticised the composition of Sanac. Some early criticisms relating to its composition were that:

- it excluded almost all South Africa's leading experts on HIV/Aids;
- key NGOs such as the Aids Consortium were not invited to be members of Sanac;
- the NGO representative, Dr Mark Ottenweller, was a foreigner with few links to NGOs;

- scientists and researchers were not recognised as a sector that should form part of Sanac;
- the medical profession, except for traditional healers, was not represented; and
- the Council was loaded with Cabinet Ministers.

In February 2000, Dr Costa Gazi, an outspoken Eastern Cape doctor, vowed to form a Shadow National Aids Council to ensure that civil society's concerns were voiced at what was regarded as the controversial process of creating Sanac.[137]

The composition of Sanac, one commentator noted, was "dictated more by exclusion – who they wanted to keep out – than by who were the best people for the job."[138] Mark Heywood asked two pertinent questions in an article in the Sowetan:

> *Why have all the experts in the science of Aids been excluded? Why has the angry voice of the activists campaigning for treatment been ignored?*[139]

Dr Gazi answered that:

> *...outspoken critics of the Minister of Health and concerned scientists have all been omitted, presumably so that the Council can work smoothly and ineffectively.*[140]

A key problem with the selection of representatives being government initiated is that it has led to a perception that pro-government persons were appointed and that it disempowers sectors from full involvement in Sanac as they cannot even determine their own sector representatives.

An appraisal of the people component of Sanac

Does Sanac's composition enable it to achieve its objectives?

It does not appear that Sanac's composition enables it to meet its objectives. It is not currently a truly multi-sectoral body, as it is dominated by government representatives. Mark Heywood argues that this has resulted in the government assuming responsibility for the response to HIV, and not developing a broad-based coalition to respond to the problem.

It is not clear why some sectors have representation on Sanac when others have been excluded. For example, the hospitality sector is represented both in the plenary and the executive; it is uncertain why it has such a significant role.

The TAC has called for Sanac to include representation from activists and scientists.[141] Ncumisa Nongogo has argued for representation from organisations representing children. The lack of private sector representation is also a glaring omission.

At the end of its first term of office, Sanac called for nominations for sector representatives for the second term of office within Sanac. It asked various sectors to hold summits and to nominate representatives. However, this process has been fraught with difficulties; for example, the PLWA community nominated two people to Sanac but both nominations were declined on the basis that the PLWA sector is in disarray.[142]

Is Sanac's size appropriate?

Both Ncumisa Nongogo and Elize Levendal say that Sanac's size makes it difficult to manage. Although there are 33 members, the meetings are frequently larger as Cabinet Ministers bring along various designated people to assist them. This results in meetings of 50 people or more, which creates problems if you are trying to facilitate participation. There is clearly a tension between the size of Sanac and the number of sectors that are represented on it. Many commentators argue that more sectors should be included on Sanac, yet it is clear that this may make it even more unmanageable.

Does Sanac have representation from vulnerable groups?

Vulnerable groups are represented on Sanac, but not in significant numbers. Thus, youth, women, the disabled and PWAs are all members of Sanac, but in each instance they only have a single representative. Thirty out of 38 members of Sanac are black.[143]

Table 5: Sector representation on Sanac

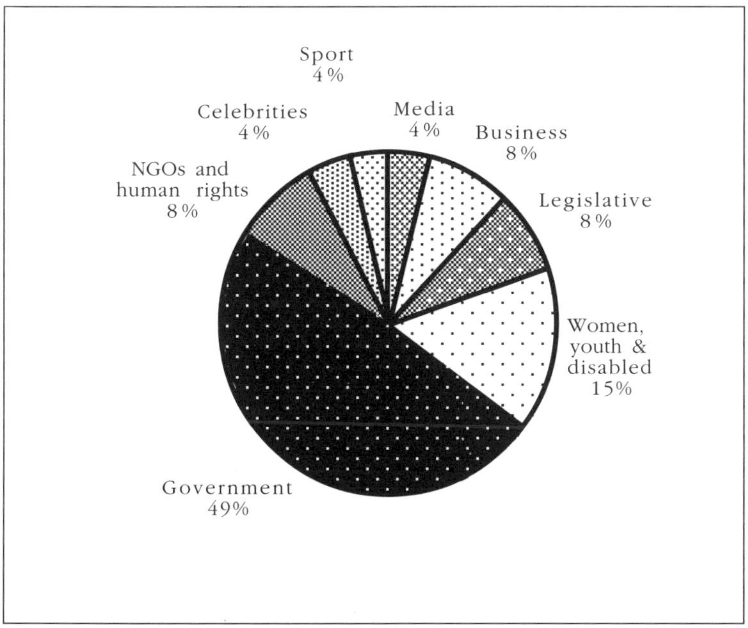

Table 6: Representation of women within Sanac

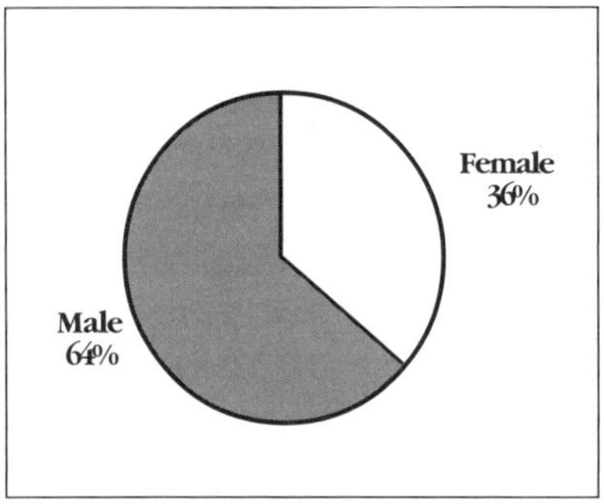

Furthermore, children are excluded although as we understand this will be rectified in Sanac's second term.[144]

An examination of the membership of Sanac shows that only 36 per cent of its members are women.

Do Sanac representatives have the necessary capacity to fulfil their duties?

It has been argued that the reason why Sanac has been so dominated by government representatives, and why the sectors have failed to make an impression, is that many of these representatives lack expertise. Conversely, it is obviously difficult to find the "ideal" representative who is both an HIV/Aids expert and can interact and represent an entire sector. It is not critical that Sanac members come from HIV/Aids organisations; rather, they should have some understanding of the issues, and Sanac should endeavour to develop their capacity on HIV/Aids.

Do Sanac representatives display leadership?

Most Sanac members have not displayed leadership within their sectors. As stated above, Sanac remains a sidelined body that has not made a significant impression on responses to HIV/Aids in South Africa. Even though Sanac has such a significant number of political leaders, it could not be argued that they are currently showing leadership on HIV/Aids within their sectors, with 26 per cent of government departments not even being in a position to report on their work. Whilst other sectors have undertaken some work, it appears to be having a limited impact. South Africa's response to HIV/Aids continues to flounder, and with regard to one of the most central issues, that of access to treatment, we have no clear plan in place.

5 Strengths and weaknesses of Sanac

Strengths

Sanac's structure is simple and clearly understood by members and stakeholders. Sanac has acknowledged that there are problems with its current structure and it is in the process of taking steps to restructure itself to bring it in line with its new role as a CCM as required by the GFATM.[145] To date, this has involved:

- appointing a consultant to review its structure;[146]
- creating an executive;
- housing the secretariat outside of the DoH;
- contracting a DFID consultant to assist it in developing a staffing plan;
- attempting to change the way in which sectoral representatives are nominated; and
- including additional sectors on Sanac.

The presence of sectoral representatives on Sanac allows for those sectors to encourage, develop and enhance the HIV/Aids response in that sector.

Best practice

The disability representative engaged with the disability sector in the following ways during 2000–2002:

- a disability summit was held from 17–18 November 2000;
- the summit made recommendations on how the DoH's Five-Year Strategic Plan on HIV/Aids could better reflect the needs of disabled persons; and
- 40 disabled persons were trained on HIV/Aids and disability in every province.

The women's sector reported that during 2000–2002:

- it had facilitated the development of Women in Partnership Against Aids (WPAA);
- provincial workshops were held on policy issues affecting women;
- provincial WPAA were launched;
- a national WPAA summit was held in March 2001;
- a strategic framework was established for WPAA;
- capacity-building workshops for 35 delegates within each province were held; and
- two capacity-building workshops were held for members of the WPAA steering committee.[147]

The potential exists for Sanac to facilitate political commitment to South Africa's response to HIV/Aids, as it is chaired by the Deputy President and has top-level representation from the Cabinet.

Sanac has reviewed its work for its first term of office and has acted on some of the recommendations made.

It has a sizeable budget for its own work and has set up a trust fund to manage its resources.

Sanac currently has a wide range of civil society sectors represented within its structures, some of whom have considerable expertise in HIV/Aids.

Weaknesses

Sanac is dominated by Cabinet Ministers, which limits the number of other sectors that can be involved in the Council.

There are no structural links between the various parts of Sanac. The technical task teams have no link with the plenary and it is not clear how the executive will interact or report back to the plenary.

There are no structural mechanisms that enable the general public to interact with Sanac and influence its agenda, and it does not have any way of interacting with sectors that are not represented on the Council. It also has limited links to other responses to HIV such as the IDC or the South African Aids Vaccine Initiative.

The predominance of government representatives on Sanac has affected the culture of the organisation, resulting in its other members feeling that they are unable to freely criticise government policies.

It does not have a strategic plan.

It has no organisational policies or procedures in place to facilitate the effective management of Sanac, or to enhance its productivity.

It has very few outputs to show for its first term of office, as few meetings were held, little interaction took place with the various sectors and it did not mobilise broader society to respond to the urgent issues relating to HIV/Aids.

It does not have systems in place to facilitate interaction between its various components; for example, between the technical task teams and the plenary.

It is difficult for a single representative to represent an entire sector. The sector is often very diverse and there may be no structures to which the representative could report.[148] It is also not possible to determine whether representatives do in fact report to their sectors. Finally, as minutes of the meetings are confidential, it is not certain what form the report backs should take.

The process of appointing sectoral representatives to Sanac is fraught with difficulties. In the first term it was government-initiated and this was problematic. The government is now supporting sectoral summits to nominate representatives for the second term; however; these have continued to be problematic. See the case study below.

Case study: Sectoral representatives

Appointing sectoral representatives for Sanac's second term was a difficult process:

The PWA nomination involved two parallel processes: one where Lucky Mazibuko was asked to nominate two persons, and the other where NAPWA organised a PWA summit. As a result, four names were sent to the Deputy President who declined them all on the basis that he was not certain which process was the most inclusive.[149]

The government is too involved in the appointment of representatives as was shown by the PWA summit, which nominated two representatives both of which were rejected by the Deputy President.[150]

The government tried to control the sectoral summits. They were, for example, opposed to the Aids Consortium facilitating the NGO summit and, as a result, it was not held.[151]

6 Recommendations

The following recommendations are made:

(1) Sanac's structure should be formalised by making it a statutory body. Mechanisms should be created within the legislation to protect its independence and its new role as a CCM. This should be undertaken with a review of the role of Sanac. It needs to establish what its core functions should be. Currently, it has too many roles and is unable to meet all the demands placed on it. Creating a statutory body also provides an opportunity to clarify roles, structure and lines of accountability, and can promote transparency. The Act must provide for formal reporting to parliament every year.

(2) The establishment of a Sanac executive should be supported. However its powers, functions and lines of accountability should be clearly stipulated. The executive should report both to Cabinet and the plenary.

(3) Steps being taken by Sanac to move the secretariat outside the DoH and to create a permanent staffing structure should be supported.

(4) The role of the technical task teams should be revisited. Currently, they are either not functioning or are functioning at a minimal level. It is however recommended that although their role needs to be refined they should not be abolished. They could act as a key technical resource to Sanac, the sectors and government departments.

(5) The implications of Sanac being a CCM need to be investigated further. Furthermore, an ad hoc task team should be set up to develop a strategy for Sanac to undertake the functions required of a CCM, such as evaluating proposals and monitoring implementation.

(6) The composition of Sanac should be revisited. Both the plenary and the executive are loaded with Cabinet Ministers who do not add significant value to the organisation. It is recommended that only three Cabinet Ministers retain their positions on Sanac, namely the ministers of health, education and social development. The "freed up" positions should be

allocated to other sectors, with the objective of increasing the representation of the following sectors without making Sanac unwieldy:
- the private sector (including financial institutions and mines);
- NGOs;
- organisations representing children;
- health professionals;
- researchers/scientists; and
- international organisations (donors and NGOs).

(7) Sanac's size should not be significantly extended; rather, other ways should be developed to ensure that sectors that are not represented on Sanac can still participate in its work. A possible solution is to follow the Ugandan example of consultations with sectors every year.

(8) The role of Sanac sector representatives should be set out in a policy document. Such a policy should cover:
- the objectives of sectoral representatives;
- how they are nominated;
- how they can represent their sector;
- who they are accountable to;
- what their responsibilities are (including report-backs and decision-making); and
- how they can access support to mobilise their sector.

(9) Resources should be made available to enable Sanac representatives to fulfil their functions.

(10) Plans to build the capacity of Sanac members should be developed, particularly advocacy skills, how to mobilise sectors and how to mainstream HIV/Aids.

(11) More formal links between the various parts of Sanac should be created. In other words, a formal link should be created between the technical task teams and the plenary. There should be a link or reporting mechanism between the executive and the plenary. There should also be formal links between Sanac and PACs.

(12) The creation of formal structures which enable the public to interact with Sanac should be supported. For example:
- allow individuals, NGOs and other organisations to make formal submissions to Sanac regarding the implementation of the Strategic Plan;
- ensure that Sanac publishes an annual report and distributes it widely;
- make minutes of meetings available to the public; and
- establish an interactive website.

(13) A strategy to develop a corporate image of Sanac should be encouraged, so as to ensure that Sanac is seen and acts as a separate body with its own identity, and not just as an extension of the DoH. This should include a clear media strategy developed by Sanac to ensure that the

Ministry of Health is not the only voice that is heard from Sanac, but that the views of other sectors are also prominent.

(14) Sanac needs to formalise its own planning and ensure that every sector develops its own plan in line with the Strategic Plan.

(15) Discussion should be entered into with donors and international organisations regarding their role in Sanac. It may be appropriate that the Ugandan model is followed and that they do not become members of Sanac, but rather a forum is set up to enable them to meet with Sanac at intervals throughout the year.

(16) Sanac's outputs should be improved by meeting regularly. PAC representatives should also attend national meetings. Meetings should focus on mobilising the sectors to become more involved in HIV/Aids. The capacity of Sanac members to undertake advocacy should be developed to enhance the response of their sectors. For example, Sanac members need to be more involved in:

- mobilising resources within every sector;
- developing capacity within sectors to respond to HIV/Aids; and
- advocating greater involvement of sectors in responses to HIV/Aids.

(17) Mobilising responses to HIV/Aids and co-ordinating efforts should be Sanac's core business. Furthermore, Sanac needs to focus its activities on the critical issues facing South Africa's responses to HIV/Aids. For example, it should currently be addressing the issue of the development of a national treatment plan.

(18) Further research should be undertaken into the effectiveness of PACs and how they can be capacitated.

(19) The capacity of Sanac to engage with the research sector should be increased by including scientists on the Council. A formal relationship should be developed with the Medical Research Council and other academic institutions, and the possibility of setting up a technical task team on research should be considered.

(20) Sanac's ability to monitor and evaluate the implementation of the Strategic Plan and the plans developed by sectors should be enhanced by developing baselines, indicators and goals.

Notes

1 Cheema GS. 2000. "Good governance: A path to poverty eradication". UNDP. Quoted in *Aids and Governance in Southern Africa; Emerging Theories and Perspectives*, Cape Town: Idasa.
2 Olowu D & Sako S (eds). 2002. *Better governance and public policy: Capacity building and democratic renewal in Africa.* New York: Kumarian Press.
3 www.worldbank.org/wbi/governance
4 www.nepad.org.ng/political_governance.htm
5 Ibid.
6 Article 25 of the UDHR states: "Everyone has the right to a standard of living adequate for the health and well being of himself and of his family, including food, clothing, housing and medical care and necessary social services, and the right to security in the event of unemployment, sickness, disability, widowhood, old age, or other lack of livelihood in circumstances beyond his control. Motherhood and childhood are entitled to special care and assistance. All children, whether born in or out of wedlock, shall enjoy the same social protection."
7 Olowu & Sako op. cit.
8 Ibid.
9 Article 21 of the UDHR stipulates: "Everyone has a right to take part in the government of his country, directly or through freely chosen representatives ... the will the people shall be the basis of the authority of government."
10 Article 2 and 7 of the UDHR speak against discrimination of all kinds and underline gender equality.
11 The APRM is a voluntary mechanism open to all member states of the African Union. States are required to sign Nepad's Declaration on Democracy, Political, Economic and Corporate Governance. They may then submit themselves to agreed parameters of good governance.
12 The World Governance Survey has crafted 30 indicators, based on the UDHR, placed in six governance dimensions for management and analytical purposes. These include freedom of association, freedom of expression, freedom from discrimination, representivity of legislatures, political competition, accountability of elected officials, political-military relations, equal treatment, equal access to justice and incorporation of international human rights norms into national laws. Cited in Olowu & Sako op. cit.
13 "Everyone, without any discrimination, has the right to equal pay for equal work." UDHR, Article 23.
14 UNDP Poverty Reduction Forum. 2000. *Zimbabwe Human Development Report.* Institute of Development Studies.
15 Ibid.
16 Ibid.
17 Ibid.
18 Ibid.
19 http://www.gov.za/yearbook/2002/landpeople.htm
20 Constitution of the Republic of South Africa, Act 108 of 1996.
21 Kenyon C, Heywood M & Conway S. 2001. "Mainstreaming HIV/Aids progress and challenges in South Africa's HIV/Aids campaign", in *South African Health Review*, Health Systems Trust.
22 Dorrington R & Johnson L. 2001. *The ingredients and impact of the HIV/Aids epidemic in South Africa and its provinces.* Durban: University of Natal Press.
23 *Mail &Guardian* 30 April–6 May 1999.

24 *Natal Witness* 18 February 2003 and the *Mail & Guardian* 21–27 February 2003.
25 Ibid.
26 Interview with Aids Consortium, 21 February 2003.
27 Hickey et al. 2003. *Budgeting for HIV/Aids in South Africa: Report on intergovernmental funding flows for an integrated response in the social sector.* Cape Town: Aids Budget Unit, Idasa, pp. 16.
28 Ibid. pp. 32.
29 Caroline Hooper-Box, *Sunday Independent* 14 March 2004.
30 The *Sunday Independent* reported that state procurement of the drugs may be delayed until July or August 2004 as arrangements had not been finalised. The *Independent* also reported that local manufacturers have been licensed to produce generic drugs, registration of drugs is being expedited by the Medicines Control Council, and health institutions countrywide are reportedly prepared to undertake the programme.
31 Ibid.
32 At the time of going to press, Gauteng became the first province to roll-out ARVs to its hospitals.
33 Cheema GS op. cit.
34 National and sector HIV/Aids policies in member states of SADC, Policy Project (2002) available from www.policyproject.com
35 These are guidelines issued by the Office of the United Nations High Commissioner for Human Rights and UNAIDS.
36 This has also been cited by the Uganda Aids Commission as a key problem.
37 National and sector HIV/Aids policies in member states of SADC, Policy Project (2002), op. cit. footnote 33.
38 http://iisd.ca/50comm/commdb/desc/d26.htm 21 February 2003.
39 www.Aidsuganda.org/uac.htm 21 February 2003.
40 Ibid.
41 Ibid.
42 These are separate meetings held between the UAC and government and the UAC and NGOs.
43 Schneider H. 1998. "The Aids policy process in South Africa," background paper for workshop on the art of policy formation: Experiences from Africa, Policy Project.
44 *Mail & Guardian* 28 January – 3 February 2000.
45 In 1997 the government was rocked by a scandal regarding an unregistered drug, Virodene. Trials on this drug, a supposed "cure" for Aids, were conducted at the University of Pretoria without ethical approval or the knowledge of the national regulator (the Medicine's Control Council). Outrage was expressed when the DoH supported a funding application to assist the researchers despite the illegal nature of their work.
46 *Mail & Guardian* 28 January – 3 February 2000.
47 Press statement obtained from http:www.polity.org.za/html/govdocs/pr/2001/pr0411.html
48 Press statement from the Office of the Deputy President, 19 February 2003.
49 *Mail & Guardian* 28 January – 3 February 2000.
50 Press statement from the Office of the Deputy President.
51 Ibid.
52 Interview with Nikko Knigge and Wayne Alexander, DoH, 19 February 2003.
53 Ibid.
54 Ibid.
55 Ibid.
56 Ibid.
57 Ibid.
58 Ibid.
59 Ibid.
60 Ibid.
61 Ibid.

62 Ibid.
63 Ibid.
64 Idasa background information on governance.
65 Ibid.
66 United Nations Development Project. 2002. *Zimbabwe Human Development Report.*
67 "A framework document for restructuring Sanac," supplied by Dr Nono Simelela, DoH.
68 National Strategic Plan 2000–2005.
69 Press release accessed on 9 January 2003 from http://www.sabcnews.co.za/Article/print_whole_story/0,1093,44465,00.html
70 Ibid.
71 Press statement issued by the Office of the Deputy President, 19 February 2003.
72 Interview with Dr Nono Simelela, Chief Director: HIV/Aids and STDs, DoH.
73 Document supplied by Dr Nono Simelela, DoH.
74 Interview with Dr Nono Simelela, DoH.
75 Aids Consortium minutes, 28 October 2002 and interview with Mr Pholokgolo Ramothwala, TAC, 6 March 2003.
76 TAC memorandum handed to Sanac on 7 October 2002, accessed from http://www.tac.org.za/newsletter/ns07_10_2002.txt
77 Ibid.
78 Interview with Ms Ncumisa Nongogo, National Trainer, Aids Legal Network.
79 Interview with Ms Sharon Ekbrahim, Aids Consortium.
80 Interview with Ms Ncumisa Nongogo, Aids Legal Network.
81 Idasa. 2000. "Finally catching up: HIV, Aids and governance in South Africa," www.idasa.org.za/m_main.php?views=2&art_id=892
82 In 2000 President Mbeki set up a Presidential Panel to investigate whether HIV causes Aids. The Nevirapine case was an action brought by the TAC to compel the government to extend its prevention of mother to child transmission of HIV programme. The case is reported as *Minister of Health and Others v Treatment Action Campaign and Others* (CCT 8/02).
83 Interview with Mr Mark Heywood, Head, Aids Law Project, 17 February 2003.
84 International Council of Aids Service Organisations. 2002. *The Global Fund to Fight Aids, TB and Malaria: Update and next steps.*
85 Sachs J. 2002. *A review of Sanac: Discussion document.*
86 Interview with Mr Mark Heywood, Aids Law Project.
87 A framework document on the restructuring of Sanac produced by an external evaluator of Sanac. See footnote 72.
88 Interview with Dr Nono Simelela, DoH. Currently, Ms Cati Vawda of the Children's Rights Centre is the children's representative on Sanac.
89 Interview with Aids Consortium.
90 Interview with Aids Law Project.
91 Dr Nono Simelela, DoH, Ms Elize Levendal, Sanac women's sector representative and Ms Ncumisa Nongogo, Aids Legal Network.
92 Interview with Dr Nono Simelela, DoH.
93 Ibid. Note that not all press statements for the meetings could be traced.
94 Interview with Ms Sharon Ekbrahim, Aids Consortium.
95 Interview with Ms Elize Levendal, women's sector representative on Sanac.
96 Interview with Ms Ncumisa Nongogo, National Trainer, Aids Legal Network.
97 *Mail & Guardian* 27 September–3 October 2002 and *Mail & Guardian* 5–11 July 2002.
98 *Mail & Guardian* 5–11 July 2002
99 Interview with Ms Sharon Ekbrahim, Aids Consortium and interview with Ms Ncumisa Nongogo, Aids Legal Network.
100 Interview with Ms Ncumisa Nongogo, Aids Legal Network.
101 Ibid.
102 Aids Consortium minutes 28 October 2002.
103 Interview with Ms Sharon Ekbrahim, Aids Consortium.

104 TAC memorandum handed to Sanac on 7 October 2002, accessed from www.tac.org.za/newsletter/ns07_10_2002.txt
105 Interview with Mr Mark Heywood, Aids Law Project.
106 Ramsey S. 2002. "Global fund makes historic first round of payments," *Lancet* (359: 1581,82).
107 The Enhancing Care Initiative (KwaZulu-Natal) (ECI) is part of a multinational care and treatment programme co-ordianted by the Harvard Aids Institute and the Francois-Xavier Bagnoud Centre for Health and Human Rights based at the Harvard School of Public Health. It aims at improving the care received by people with HIV or Aids in resource-constrained countries through facilitating policy and health-care delivery in developing countries. It saw itself as ideally placed to submit a proposal to the fund. It was a university, government and civil society partnership. It had already undertaken two years of community research involving 795 HIV/Aids-infected patients and 456 health-care providers within 70 health institutions in KwaZulu-Natal. Furthermore, its proposal had the support of all these stakeholders, including the provincial DoH.
108 Heywood M. 2002. "Human rights and the Global Fund: South Africa stumbles at its first hurdle," *Aids Amaryllises Africa*, October/November.
109 *Mail & Guardian*, 27 September–3 October 2002.
110 Since the time of writing, the revised proposal was submitted and received funding and a number of projects have started implementing their programmes. Personal correspondence with Dr Robert Pawinski, ECI, 4 May 2004.
111 Interview with Dr Nono Simelela, DoH.
112 This took place in February 2002.
113 Sachs J op. cit.
114 Interview with Dr Nono Simelela, DOH.
115 Aids Consortium minutes, 28 October 2002.
116 Press statement issued by the Office of the Deputy President, 19 February 2003.
117 Interview with Ms Ncumnisa Nongogo, Aids Legal Network.
118 Interview with Dr Nono Simelela, DoH.
119 This ran from April 2001 to March 2002.
120 This ran from April 2002 to March 2003.
121 This runs from April 2003 to March 2004. Information on the Sanac budget was obtained from www.doh.gov.za
122 Interview with Ms Ncumisa Nongogo, Aids Legal Network.
123 Interview with Mr Mark Heywood, Aids Law Project. Mr Pholokgolo Ramothwala of the TAC argued that if Sanac was to become a CCM it would need to ensure that its decisions were binding.
124 Interview with Ms Ncumisa Nongogo, Aids Legal Network.
125 Interview with Mark Heywood, Aids Law Project, TAC Memorandum, 17 October 2002.
126 Interview with Mr Phologolo Ramothwala, TAC.
127 *Mail & Guardian*, 27 September–3 October 2002.
128 Press release accessed on the 9 January 2003 from www.sabcnews.co.za/Article/print_whole_story/0,1093,144465,00.html
129 Press statement released by the Office of the Deputy President, 19 February 2003.
130 Personal communication between Dr Sachs and Ms Kitty Barrett Grant, 20 February 2003.
131 A framework document on the restructuring of Sanac. See footnotes 72 and 86.
132 This included significant departments and bodies such as the Departments of Labour, Defence and Health.
133 Note reports were allowed to list more than one activity.
134 A framework document on the restructuring of Sanac, op.cit. footnote 127.
135 March 2000.
136 AIDS Consortium minutes, 28 October 2002.
137 *Mail & Guardian*, 4–10 February 2000. It does not appear that this initiative ever got off the ground.
138 *Mail & Guardian*, 28 January–3 February 2000.

139 *Aids Bulletin*, March 2000.
140 Ibid.
141 *Mail & Guardian*, 27 September–3 October 2002.
142 Interview with Mr Mark Heywood, Aids Law Project, 17 February 2003.
143 Interview with Dr Nono Simelela, DoH.
144 Interview with Dr Nono Simelela, DoH.
145 Press statement issued by the Office of the Deputy President, 19 February 2003.
146 Dr J Sachs was appointed to undertake a review of Sanac during 2002.
147 Dr J Sachs. *A review of Sanac: Discussion document*.
148 Interview with Ms Elize Levendal, women's sector representative on Sanac.
149 Interview with Dr Nono Simelela, DoH.
150 Interview with Ms Pholokgolo Ramothwala, TAC.
151 Interview with Mr Mark Heywood, Aids Law Project.
152 *AIDS Bulletin*, March 2000.
153 Information received from the TAC memorandum to Sanac dated 7 October 2002.
154 Interview with Mr Mark Heywood, Head, Aids Law Project, 17 February 2003.
155 Interview with Ms Ncumisa Nongogo, National Trainer, Aids Legal Network.
156 Press statement issued by the Chairperson of Sanac, issued on 19 February 2003.

Appendix 1:

People interviewed in the preparation of this report

Interviews were held with, amongst others:

- treatment activists;
- Sanac members – sector representatives;
- Aids activists in NGOs; and
- government department officials

List of key people interviewed:

Mark Heywood, Aids Law Project and Treatment Action Campaign
Ncumisa Nongogo, Aids Legal Network and member of Sanac
Sharon Ekbrahim, Aids Consortium
Nikko Knigge, Department of Health, Directorate of HIV/Aids and STDs
Wayne Alexander, Department of Health, Directorate of HIV/Aids and STDs
Nono Simelela, Department of Health, Chief Directorate of HIV/Aids and STDs
Colley Carey, HIV/Aids Co-ordinator, Department of Land Affairs
Elize Levedal, women's sector representative, Sanac
Pholokgolo Ramothwala, Treatment Action Campaign
Rose Smart, HIV/Aids consultant
Johnny Sachs, Consultant
Robert Pawinski, Enhancing Care Initiative, KwaZulu-Natal

Appendix 2:

Institutional appraisal of key governance institutions relating to HIV and Aids in South Africa

1. Background

1.1 Explanation of research project and aims, objectives and format of the interview
1.2 Information on interviewee, for example:
1.3 Position
1.4 Functions
1.5 Do they want their name reflected in the report?
1.6 Are they speaking in an official or unofficial capacity?

2. External environment and context

2.1 Describe the political environment within which Sanac works
2.2 Does the current legislative/policy framework on HIV/Aids allow for all persons, including the poor, to participate in policy making?
2.3 Are basic HIV/Aids services being provided to all people?
2.4 Does the legislative and policy framework protect the rights of persons affected by HIV/Aids?
2.5 Does national government "lead" or provide leadership on HIV/Aids?
2.6 Are there any economic, social or financial factors that influence HIV/Aids policies?

3. Structure

3.1 Describe the structure of Sanac
3.2 Is there an up-to-date organisation chart?
3.3 Do members have a clear idea of the structure?
3.4 Does it have an executive? If yes, what is its function?
3.5 Does it have a secretariat? If yes, what is its function?
3.6 Roles and responsibilities
3.7 What is the role/function of Sanac?
   3.7.1 In policy documents, etc.
   3.7.2 In the interviewees opinion
3.8 In the view of other stakeholders
   3.8.1 Who determines its functions?
3.9 Is there a business plan/strategic plan?
   3.9.1 Who developed the business plan?

3.9.2 How was it developed?
3.10 In its functions, how does it relate to other structures?
3.10.1 IDC provincial
3.10.2 IDC's broader political structures
3.10.3 Implementers such as government departments
3.10.4 Funding organisations, broader organisations such as civil society/private sector
3.11 Who takes decisions (Sanac or DoH/Cabinet) regarding HIV/Aids strategy?
3.12 Who takes decisions regarding HIV/Aids funding? Who takes decisions regarding HIV/Aids implementation?
3.13 What are the problems it has in carrying out its functions?
3.14 What should Sanac's functions be (the ideal)?

4. Accountability

4.1 Who is Sanac accountable to?
4.2 Are there problems with this? How could it be improved?
4.3 Are minutes of meetings kept and distributed?
4.4 Are minutes put to the meeting for confirmation of accuracy and signed as a fair reflection of the meeting?
4.5 Are members asked to report back on matters arising? To whom?
4.6 Can the public obtain access to the minutes? How?
4.6 Describe how a national institution such as Sanac should be accountable
4.7 Lines of control/reporting
4.8 To whom does Sanac report? Is there any reporting mechanism for reporting activities of Sanac (e.g. annual report)?
4.9 How are decisions of Sanac made known to broader stakeholders?
4.10 Interface with other stakeholders
4.11 How can non-members participate in Sanac?
4.12 How can the concerns of non-members be heard at Sanac?
4.13 Is there any provision for the concerns of vulnerable groups (such as women and children) to be heard at Sanac?
4.14 Describe current levels of participation by non-members
4.15 Describe how SANAC should be making itself accessible (the ideal)

5. Culture

5.1 Attitudes
5.2 What are the attitudes of members of Sanac regarding its role and functions?
5.3 Is Sanac independent?
5.4 Values

5.5 What are the organisational values/norms or culture of Sanac (e.g. are all decisions made on a consensus basis or by majority vote)?
5.6 Describe current levels and forms of participation by members
5.7 What are barriers to participation? How could it be improved?
5.8 Management style
5.9 What is the role of the Chairperson of Sanac?
5.10 How are decisions of Sanac meetings taken?
5.11 Are there different levels of decision-making?
5.12 Behaviour
5.13 Are the political leaders of Sanac able to:
  5.13.1 Mobilise political commitment to HIV/Aids?
  5.13.2 Provide strategic direction to HIV/Aids?
  5.13.3 Mobilise implementation of HIV/Aids responses in their sectors, departments, etc?

6. Systems and processes

6.1 Planning
6.2 Does it have an annual/bi-annual planning process?
6.3 Who is involved in planning?
6.4 What are the outputs of the planning process?
6.5 How and by whom are these used?
6.6 Are budgets developed on the basis of plans developed this way?
6.7 Financial management
6.8 How is Sanac funded?
6.9 What is the size of its budget?
6.10 Is information available on how the budget is spent?
6.11 Is the whole budget spent every year?
6.12 What happens to funds that are not spent?
6.13 Is any funding received from donors?
6.14 How is this used?
6.15 What are the donor objectives?
6.16 Are members paid for their time on Sanac?
6.17 What is the proportion of funding spent on staffing/members' costs, as compared to costs relating to its functions?
6.18 In funding projects, is money spent equitably and in a manner that is pro-poor and benefits marginalised groups?
6.19 In practice, how does Sanac award contracts/tenders, etc?
6.20 Are policies in place to prevent corruption or abuse of funding (e.g. policies preventing Sanac members from personally benefiting from contracts)?
6.21 Does an internal audit system exist?
6.22 What influence does Sanac have over government budget allocations? Does it guide/advise government before the budget speech?

6.23 Management information
6.24 How (process) is Sanac monitored or evaluated?
6.25 Has it ever been evaluated?
6.26 Are the results available?
6.27 Personnel
6.28 Does Sanac have staff working for it? If yes, describe number and tasks
6.29 Work processes
6.30 Who determines issues to be placed on the agenda of Sanac meetings?
6.31 Who can Sanac bind through its decisions (itself, other stakeholders; i.e. internal and external accountability)?
6.32 Are tasks delegated?
6.33 Do members report back on tasks?
6.34 How do outsiders view decision-making?
6.35 Can they describe instances of poor decision-making?
6.36 How does Sanac determine productivity? Does non-attendance at meetings result in a sanction?

7. People

7.1 Numbers
7.2 How many members does Sanac have?
7.3 What is the race, gender and disability breakdown of membership?
7.4 Composition
7.5 Describe the composition of Sanac
7.6 Who determined the composition?
7.7 How were people appointed?
7.8 What political leaders are represented on Sanac?
7.9 Is it a manageable size?
7.10 Is it representative?
7.11 Are sectors left out?
7.12 Are sectors sufficiently represented (e.g. is each sector given one place)?
7.13 What vulnerable groups are represented on Sanac (women, children, rural people)?
7.14 How do sectors determine their representatives?
7.15 Do sector representatives report back to their constituency?
7.16 How should Sanac be composed (ideal)?
7.17 Skills
7.18 Do members of Sanac have sufficient skills?
7.19 Are resources devoted to capacity development?
7.20 Knowledge
7.21 Do Sanac members have accurate, up-to-date information on HIV/Aids?
7.22 Is this knowledge reflected in their decision-making?
7.23 Leadership

7.24 What is the leadership role of Sanac itself, in relation to other institutions, processes, departments, etc? Please describe?
7.25 Does Sanac fulfil its leadership role? Describe successes and failures
7.26 How could it be improved?
7.27 Does Sanac leadership/executive provide internal leadership?

8. General

8.1 Describe strengths
8.2 Is it effective? Does it carry out its mandate?
8.3 Can you give an example of its successes in carrying out its functions?
8.4 What are its successes?
8.5 Describe its weaknesses
8.6 Is it able to fulfil its mandate?
8.7 Is it sustainable?

Appendix 3:

Members of Sanac as appointed by the president in January 2000 for the first term of office[152]

1. Deputy President, Jacob Zuma (Chair)
2. Dr M Tshabalala-Msimang, Minister of Health
3. Prof. K Asmal, Minister of Education
4. Dr ZS Skweyiya, Minister of Social Development
5. Ms AT Didiza, Minister of Agriculture
6. Mr D Omar, Minister of Transport (now deceased)
7. Mr M Mdladlana, Minister of Labour
8. Mr T Manuel, Minister of Finance
9. Mr FS Mufamadi, Minister of Provincial and Local Government
10. Mr MGP Lekota, Minister of Defence
11. Ms P Mlambo-Ngeuka, Minister of Minerals and Energy
12. Mr BM Skosana, Minister of Correctional Services
13. Mr A Omar, Government Communication and Information Service
14. Dr SA Nkomo, Chairperson of the Health Portfolio Committee
15. Ms L Jacobs, Chairperson of the Select Committee Social Services
16. Mr Bongani Khumalo, business representative
17. Mr Lucky Mazibuko, People Living with HIV and Aids
18. Dr Mark Ottenweller, NGOs' representative
19. Rev Cedric Mayson, faith-based organisations' representative
20. Mr Zwelinzima Vavi, trade unions' representative
21. Ms Elise Levendal, women's groups' representative
22. Mr Sizwe Shezi, youth groups' representative
23. Mr Majjore Lehasa, traditional healers' representative
24. Chief M Mzimela, traditional leaders' representative
25. Ms N Nongongo, legal and human rights' representative
26. Ms H Bogopare, disabled people's representative
27. Ms N Gongxeka, celebrities' representative
28. Mr R Moeti, sport bodies' representative
29. Ms D Cooper, media representative
30. Dr S Dhlomo, local government representative
31. Ms N Nhlapo, hospitality industry representative

The following changes have been made to this list since January 2000:

1. Mr BS Ngubane, Minister of Arts, Culture, Science and Technology.
2. Dr Ngculu, Chairperson of the Health Portfolio Committee (replaced Dr Nkomo).

3. Ms H Bogopane (sector unknown).
4. Mr T Ndoro, National Association of People Living with HIV and AIDS (replaced Mr L Mazibuko who resigned).[153]
5. Mr Bongani Khumalo, representing business, has resigned and has not been replaced.
6. Two more labour representatives have been added, but their names were not available.[154] An additional PLWA representative has been added, but his or her name was not available at the time of writing this report.[155]

Appendix 4:

List of members of the Sanac excutive for the first term of office:

1. Dr M Tshabala-Msimang, Minister of Health
2. Ms T Didiza, Minister of Agriculture
3. Mr D Omar, Minister of Transport (now deceased)
4. Mr M Mdladlana, Minister of Labour
5. Ms N Madlala Routledge, Deputy Minister of Defence
6. Mr T Doro, NAPWA
7. Mrs E Levendal, women's sector
8. Ms L Nhlapo, hospitality sector
9. Ms J Pekane, Cosatu[156]

Appendix 5:

Governance & Aids National Seminar (Towards Treatment, Care & Support)

Attendance register
Venue: Burgers Park Hotel
Date: 27 November 2003

Name & Surname	Organisation	Postal address	Telephone	Fax	e-mail
1.Catherine Sozi	UNAIDS	351 Schoeman St Box 6541 Pretoria 0001	082 9092639 012-3548484	012-3548451	e-mail: csozi@un.org.za
2. C.Vidah Mayana	Planned Parenthood Association of S.A	P.O. Box 2655 North End Port Elizabeth 6056	082 8210119 041-4872672	041-4844083	e-mail: ppaec@wn.apc.org
3. Sesupo Makaole-Nene	Department of Health (Sanac)	P/Bag X828 Pretoria 0001	012-3120131	012-3123115	e-mail: nenes@health.gov.za
4. Rita Muyambo	Project Support Group (PSG)	P.O. Box 1251 Bethal 2310	072-6381266 017-6476840	017-6473692	e-mail: rmuyambo@gmx
5. Ann Strode	University of Natal School of Law	P/Bag X01 Scottsville 3209	082 5733920 033-2605731	033-2605015	e-mail: strodeA@nu.ac.za
6. Zini Godden	Netherlands Embassy	P.O. Box 117 Pretoria 0001	012-3443910	012-3440781	e-mail: zini.godden@minbuza.nl
7. Stella T Ndabeni	Eastern Cape Aids Council	Global Life Building Cnr. Phalo Avenue & Bisho Umtata	082 9214948 040-6351590	040-6351571	e-mail: stella-ecac@ecsecc.org
8. Belarmino Manjate	Positive Women's Network	Postnet X21 Suite 159 Sunnyside 0132 Pretoria	083 3713276 012-3920500	012-3202414/5	e-mail: bmanjate@pwn.org.za

Name & Surname	Organisation	Postal address	Telephone	Fax	e-mail
9. Vuyani Jacobs	Treatment Action Campaign	34 Main Road Muizenberg, Cape Town 8001	0824209475 021-7883507	021-7883266	e-mail: vuyani@tac.org.za
10. Luann Hatane	Western Cape Networking Aids Community of SA	P.O. Box 6358 Roggebaai 8012	0832530886 021-4254308	021-4218754	e-mail: director@wc-nacosa.co.za
11. Duduzile Chandiwana	UNDP Regional Project on HIV and Development	P.O. Box 6541 Pretoria 0001	012-3699934	012-3487688	e-mail: dudu.chandiwana@undp.org
12. Innocent Modisaotsile	SADC Health	P/Bag X828 Pretoria 0001	0828504148 012-3120338	012-3123150	e-mail: modisi@health.gov.za
13. Felicity Hatendi	Zimbabwe Consultant	P.O. Box 268 WGT Harare, Zimbabwe	09263 4 309728		e-mail: fhatendi@ecoweb.co.zw
14. Manasa Dzirikure	SADC	P/Bag X828 Pretoria 0001	0825666825 012-3120365	012-3123150	e-mail: dzirim@health gov.za
15. Bongani Nkosi	Centre for the Study of Aids (CSA)	Cnr. Lunnon & Tindal Street University of Pretoria Pretoria 0002	0834720845 012-4204484	012-4204395	e-mail: bnkosi@postino.up.ac.za
16. Sphindile Magwaza	Development Co-operation Ireland	P.O. Box 4174 Pretoria 0001	0832188718 012-3425062	012-3424752	e-mail: sphindile.magwaza@iveagh.irlgvv-.ie
17. Xoli Mahlalela	Equity Project/Eastern Cape Aids Council	P.O. Box 1575 Garsfontein 0060	0833067707 012-3446117	012-3446115	e-mail: xolim@equityproject.co.za

Name & Surname	Organisation	Postal address	Telephone	Fax	e-mail
19. Ana Monteiro	Centre for African Studies	P O Box 8828 Bachbrecht, Windhoek Namibia	09258 1 480826	09258 1 49896	monteirolluk@yahoo.co.uk
20. M. Molapo	CSIR	P O Box 91230 Auckland Park Johannesburg 2006	011-3580222	011-4823267	mmolapo@csir.co.za
21. Robyn	Idasa	P O Box 56950 Arcadia 0007	012-3920500	012-3202415	robyn@idasa.org.za
22. Marietjie Myburg	Idasa	P O Box 56950 Arcadia 0007	012-3920500	012-3202415	marietjie@idasa.org.za
23. Kondwani Chirambo	Idasa	P O Box 56950 Arcadia 0007	012-3920500	012-3202415	kondwani@idasa.org.za
24. Mary Caesar	Idasa	P O Box 56950 Arcadia 0007	012-3920500	012-3202415	mary@idasa.org.za
25. Beate Jaschik	Idasa	P O Box 56950 Arcadia 0007	012-3920500	012-3202415	beate@idasa.org.za
26. Vas Naicker	Idasa	P O Box 56950 Arcadia 0007	012-3920500	012-3202415	vas@idasa.org.za